AF879959

Physeo

TABLE OF CONTENTS

We would like to extend a special thanks to the following individuals who have spent many hours tutoring, guiding and consulting this work, making Physeo possible

Paloma F Cariello, MD, MPH
Assistant Professor
Division of Infectious Diseases
University of Utah School of Medicine
Salt Lake City, UT

Karen Eilbeck, Ph.D.
Professor
Biomedical Informatics
University of Utah

Vicente Planelles, Ph.D.
Professor
Division of Microbiology and Immunology
Department of Pathology
University of Utah School of Medicine
Salt Lake City, UT

Carol Foote
MD Candidate Class of 2021
University of Utah Schoold of Medicine
Salt Lake City, UT

David Ortiz
MD Candidate Class of 2021
University of Utah Schoold of Medicine
Salt Lake City, UT

Naveen Rathi
MD Candidate Class of 2021
University of Utah Schoold of Medicine
Salt Lake City, UT

PSYCHIATRY

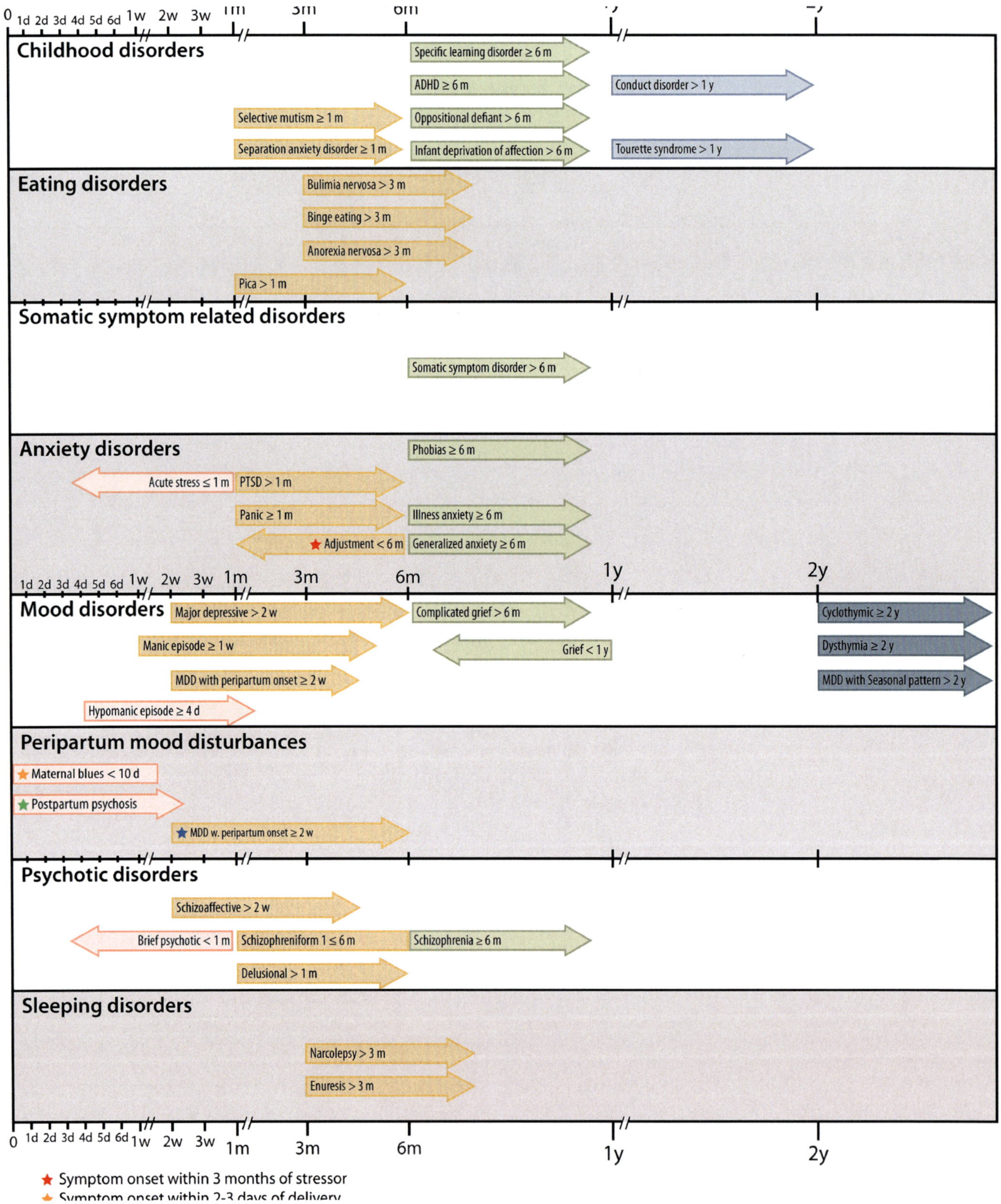

FIGURE 19.1.1 - Psychiatric Overview Figure

I. Overview
   A. Infant deprivation of affection
   B. Child abuse
   C. Child neglect
   D. Vulnerable child syndrome

II. Infant Deprivation of Affection
   A. Infants have a physiological and psychological need for affection
   B. Deprivation effects
      1. Reactive attachment disorder and poor development of trust
      2. Failure to thrive
      3. Poor language and social development
   C. Infant deprivation vs child neglect
   D. Lack of affection vs lack of basic needs

III. Infant Deprivation: Long-term Effects
   A. Long-term deprivation (>6 months) can result in permanent psychiatric problems
   B. Extreme cases can result in death

IV. Burns and Bruises
   A. Locations
      1. TEN4: Torso, Ears, Neck folds in children <4-years-old
   B. Patterns
      1. Well-defined marks from specific objects are red flags
      2. Buckle, board, spatula, stick/whip, grid, cigarette, immersion
   C. Mongolian spots

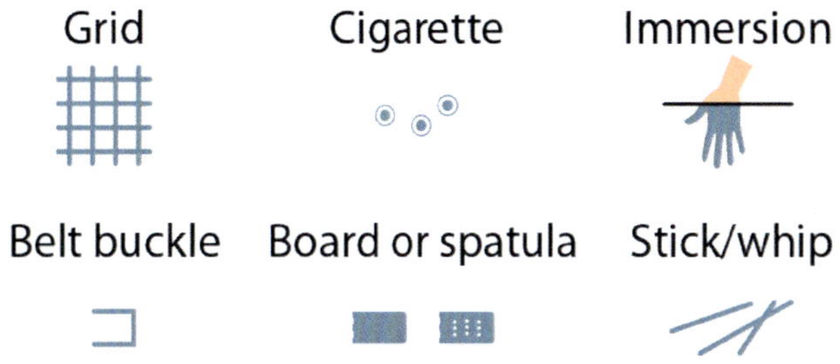

FIGURE 19.1.2 - Child Abuse Patterns

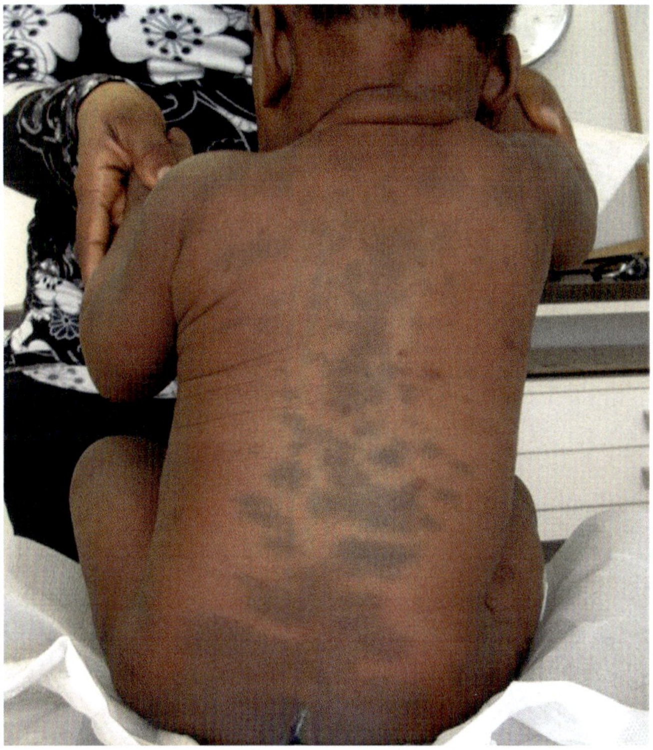

FIGURE 19.1.3 - Mongolian Spots

Abuse Type	Physical Clues	Historical Clues	Abuser	Epidemiology
Physical	- Burns and bruises - Fractures - Subdural hematomas, retinal detachment or retinal hemorrhage	- Unexplained injuries - Age-inappropriate injuries - Caregiver denies injury - Caregiver delays seeking care	- Biological mother or primary caregiver	- Most common victims: Infants
Sexual	- Physical signs may be absent - STIs - UTIs - Trauma to the oral, anal, or genital regions	- Inappropriate sexual behavior/ knowledge based on age	- Adult male known to victim	- Most common victims: Prepubescent girls (9-12) - Results in high rates of PTSD, depression, and suicidality
Emotional	- Physical signs are usually absent	- Avoids caretaker - Clingy or attach readily to strangers - Prone to emotional outbursts and aggression - Vague/unexplained somatic symptoms	- Parent or caregiver	- Results in high rates of psychiatric illness or delay in social, emotional and developmental skills

TABLE 19.1.1 - Child Abuse

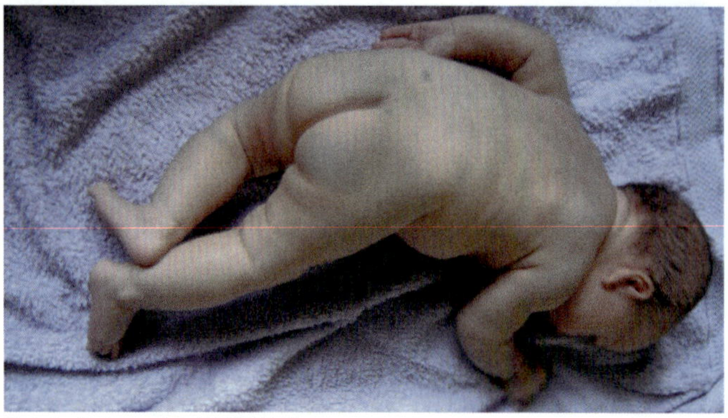

Photo Credit: Geowombats (CC BY-SA 2.0)

FIGURE 19.1.4 - Mongolian Spots

V. Fractures
   A. Red flags
      1. Adjacent rib fractures
      2. Multiple fractures at different stages of healing

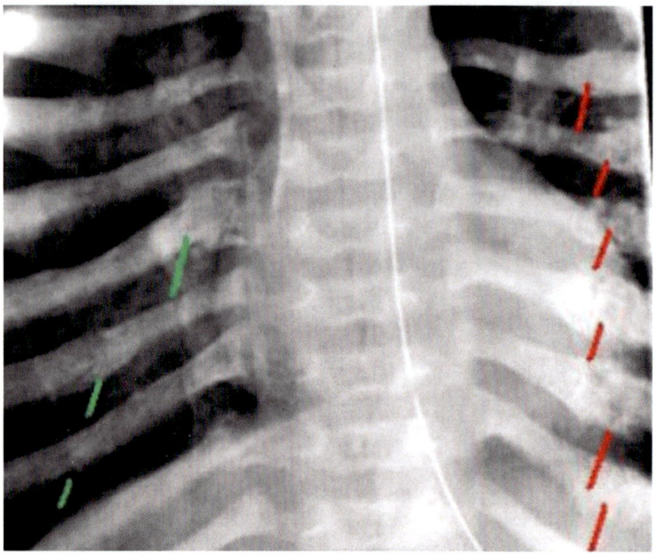

Photo Credit: National Institute of Health [Public domain]

FIGURE 19.1.5 - Chest X-Ray Showing Adjacent Rib Fractures

VI. Abusive Head Trauma
   A. Subdural hematoma
   B. Retinal detachment
   C. Retinal hemorrhage

VII. Emotional Abuse
   A. Definition: The degrading of a child's self-esteem or emotional well-being.
      1. Verbal or behavioral
      2. Involves constant criticism, intimidation, withholding affection, humiliation, refusing to communicate, belittling, berating, and even rejecting or isolating a child

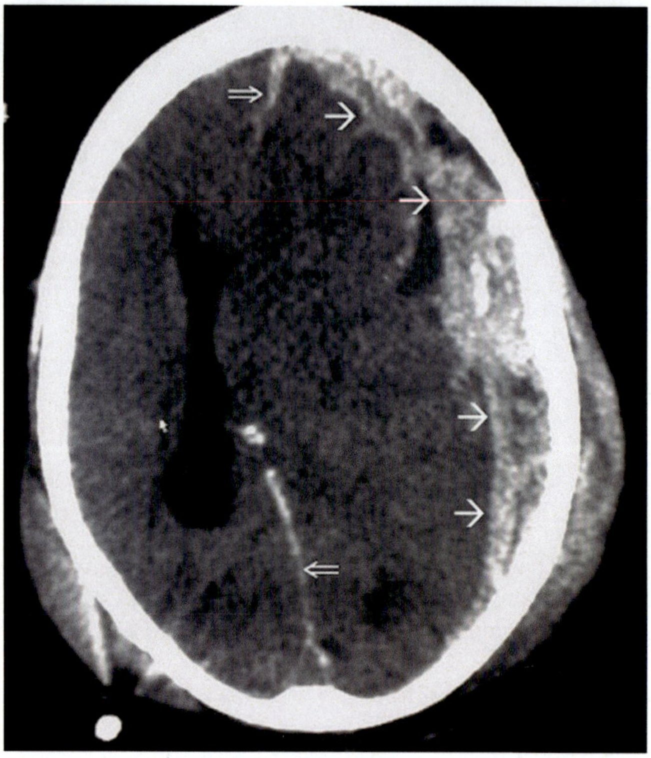

Photo Credit: 2007-06-24 17:16 Glitzy queen00 [Public domain]

FIGURE 19.1.6 - Subdural Hematoma

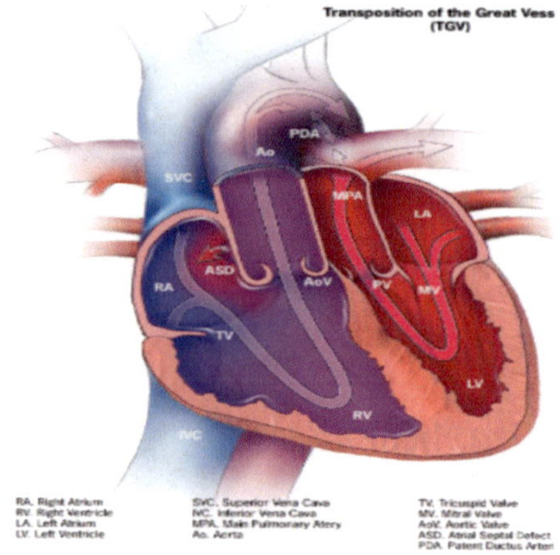

Photo Credit: www.flickr.com/photos/hobbs_images/2590555768/in/photostream/

FIGURE 19.1.7 - Retinal Hemorrhage

VIII. Child Neglect
   A. Most common form of child abuse
   B. Failure to provide adequate shelter, food, education, supervision, affection, and medical or dental care
   C. Evidence of neglect ranges from malnutrition to psychosocial deficits

IX. Vulnerable Child Syndrome
   A. Opposite of child neglect: characterized by overprotective parenting
   B. Risk factors
      1. Serious illness or near-death experience of the child
   C. Parental worry leads to overuse of medical services and missed school

REVIEW QUESTIONS

1. What's the difference between infant deprivation and child neglect?

   - **Child neglect deals with children of any age and the failure to provide them with the necessary components of a functional life - shelter, food, affection, education, and supervision. Kids who have been neglected often appear unkempt, malnourished, withdrawn, or physically and emotionally stunted.**
   - Infant deprivation deals specifically with infants and affection. The effects of infant deprivation are pretty much the same (poor growth and development and poor development of trust) but the difference is that infant deprivation deals specifically with a lack of love or affection during early development that led to the physiological and psychological problems later on.

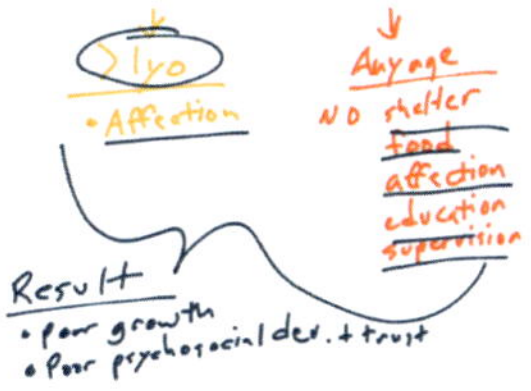

2. A 4-year-old girl is brought to the physician for her annual check-up from foster care. She was abandoned by her parents at the age of 3 months. The patient is extremely friendly and openly greets the medical staff. She plays with with her dolls during physical examination and hugs the physician afterwards. What are the similarities and differences between this patient's condition and reactive attachment disorder?

   - **While disinhibited social engagement disorder is characterized by extreme friendliness and openness to strangers, reactive attachment disorder present with social withdrawal, sadness, and fear. This 4-year-old girl presents for her annual check-up from foster care.**
   - She was abandoned by her parents at the age of 3 months. Therefore, she has experienced child neglect.
   - She is extremely friendly and openly greets the medical staff.
   - She plays with with her dolls during physical examination and hugs the physician afterwards.
   - Open friendliness and active social interactions with strangers in the context of child neglect suggest the diagnosis of disinhibited social engagement disorder.
   - Child neglect, abuse, or trauma can potentially lead to either disinhibited social engagement disorder or reactive attachment disorder.

3. An 11-year-old girl living with her mother and aunt comes into the office due to bad stomach aches. She says that they have been going on for over a month now and it hurts to urinate. She is timid and avoids eye contact with the physician. During the interview the mom states that they live alone but that both she and her sister have boyfriends that frequently spend the night. Urinalysis is performed and WBC counts are within normal ranges. What is an appropriate next step in treating the child?

   A. Assess for STI
   B. Urine culture
   C. Interview parent alone
   D. Skeletal survey
   E. Toxicology screen

   - **The correct answer is A.**
   - This young girl is likely the victim of sexual abuse. She is in the high risk age range (9-12-years-old) and there are two males that are in frequent contact with the family. She has signs of sexual abuse and an appropriate next step would be to assess for the signs of abuse, possible pregnancy, or STI.
   - B is incorrect because the urinalysis was already performed which makes UTI unlikely.
   - So a Urine culture wouldn't be very informative.
   - Interviewing the parent alone isn't standard procedure in cases of suspected abuse.
   - However, interviewing the child alone may be appropriate since abused children will often not disclose abuse during the interview with the parent in the room.
   - A skeletal survey is indicated in cases of suspected physical abuse because it scans all bones of the body for fractures.
   - This case does not have any red flags indicative of physical abuse so this test would not be necessary.
   - Finally, this girl doesn't have signs or symptoms of drug use or poisoning and so a toxicology screen wouldn't fit here.

Psychiatry | Section 2: Childhood Behavior & Anxiety Disorders

Disorder	Time	Key Features	Treatment	Memory Hooks
Conduct disorder	≥ 3 symptoms for ≥ 1 year with 1 symptom lasting for ≥ 6 months	- Pattern of behavior that violates the basic human rights of others and breaks societal norms (theft, aggression, cruel acts) - After age 18: antisocial personality disorder	- CBT	CD = Criminal Deeds
Oppositional defiant disorder	≥ 6 months	- Angry, irritable mood, argumentative/defiant behavior to authority figures, often vindictive - No criminal actions	- CBT	ODD = Openly Defiant and vinDictive
Disruptive mood dysregulation disorder	Onset: < 10 years-old	- Pattern of explosive outbursts of anger (≥3x/ week) - May be verbal or physical - Disproportionate for the situation - Incongruent with developmental stage	- Antipsychotics - Stimulants	DMDD = TNT explosive tantrums
Selective mutism	≥ 1 month	- An anxiety disorder - Onset before 5-years-old - Symptoms last for >1 month - Normal language and speech abilities - Only silent in certain situations → impaired functioning in school or social settings due to silence	- CBT - Family/play therapy - SSRIs	Mute for a month
Separation anxiety disorder	≥ 1 month	- An anxiety disorder characterized by excessive worry surrounding an attachment figure (being separated or harm coming to the figure) - Nightmares - Nausea or headache in anticipation of separation - Factitious complaints possible to avoid separation	- CBT - Family/play therapy	SAD to leave

TABLE 19.1.2 - Childhood Behavior & Anxiety Disorders

I. Cognitive Behavioral Therapy
   A. Purpose: help patients identify/correct distorted, maladaptive beliefs
      1. Used to treat many different psychiatric conditions
   B. Techniques:
      1. Education
      2. Relaxation exercises
      3. Coping skills training
      4. Stress management
      5. Assertiveness training

REVIEW QUESTIONS

?

1. A 7-year old boy is brought to the clinic by his mother due to behavioral issues. She states that for the last year he has been consistently talking back to his parents and teachers. She states that he behaves very differently and more appropriately when interacting with his friends. However, whenever she or his father asks him to do something, he gets overly angry and refuses to do it. What is the most likely diagnosis?

    - **Based on this boy's argumentative behavior towards authority figures, like parents and teachers, for over 6 months he most likely has oppositional defiant disorder.**
    - This boy is brought in for behavioral issues, mainly talking back to his parents and teachers.
    - He gets overly angry when asked to do anything by his parents and he usually refuses to do what is asked of him.
    - However when interacting with his friends he has no issue.
    - It is important to differentiate this disorder from conduct disorder.
    - On of the keys in separating the two is how the patient acts towards peers of their own age.
    - Those with conduct disorder, show no empathy and violate the rights of anyone, including their peers.
    - Those with oppositional defiant disorder, only have issues with authority figures, not typically their own peers.

2. A 5-year old boy is brought to the clinic because his mother is worried about his behavior. He started kindergarten 6 weeks ago and throws tantrums whenever his mother drops him off. He states that occasionally he has nightmares about his mother forgetting him at school even though it has never happened. His mother states that over the past week he has been trying to get out of going to school by acting like he has a cough or is nauseous. Which of the following is the best treatment option for this boy?

    A. SSRI
    B. Family or play therapy
    C. Stimulants
    D. Antipsychotics

    - **The correct answer is B.**
    - This young boy presents due to outbursts or tantrums whenever his mother drops him off at kindergarten.
    - He reports nightmares about the situation.
    - He also engages in making factitious complaints to avoid his mother leaving him at school.
    - Based on these symptoms, this boy most likely has separation anxiety disorder.
    - This is best treated with either CBT or family/play therapy, thus making answer choice B correct.
    - Answer choice A is incorrect because SSRIs can be utilized in selective mutism, not separation anxiety.
    - Answer choices C & D are incorrect because stimulants and antipsychotics can be used in disruptive mood dysregulation disorder, not separation anxiety.

Disease	Time	Key Features	Treatment
ADHD	≥ 6 months	Onset: <12 years old; diagnose by identifying symptoms of hyperactivity, impulsivity and inattention; more common in boys; normal intelligence; many comorbid conditions possible (tourette, mood disorders, behavioral disorders, specific learning disorder)	Stimulants, CBT, α_2-agonists
Specific learning disorder	> 6 months	Inability to learn a specific school subject (reading, writing, math, etc.) despite focused help; normal intelligence, low test scores in particular subject; rule out other primary causes (hearing/vision loss, autism, ADHD) with screening and history	Counselling, tutoring, after school activities
Intellectual disability	Daily function	Global deficits of intellectual and adaptive skills; problems with conceptual, practical, and social skills that affect daily living	Family support, special education, skill development
Autism spectrum disorder		Onset during early childhood; characterized by social deficits, insistence on routines, altered sensory perception, restricted or repetitive patterns of behavior; savants	Educational and behavioral therapy

TABLE 19.1.3 - Childhood and Early-Onset Disorders

I. Attention-Deficit Hyperactivity Disorder (ADHD)
   A. More common in boys
   B. Two types of symptoms
      1. Hyperactivity and impulsivity
      2. Inattention

II. ADHD: Hyperactivity and Impulsivity
   A. Excessive talking, restless, interrupts others, constantly moving
   B. ↑ impulsivity →↑ risk of substance use disorders
   C. Outward signs of hyperactivity and impulsivity decrease with age

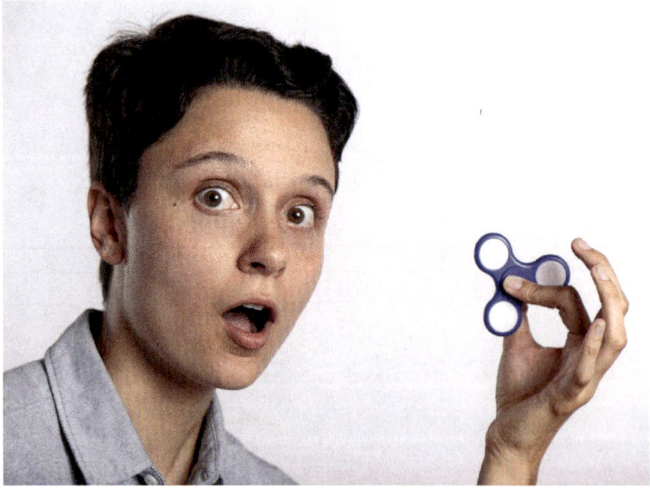

Photo Credit: Pixabay

FIGURE 19.1.8 - Hyperactivity & Impulsivity

III. ADHD: Inattention
   A. Normal intelligence but may struggle in school
   B. Inattention
      1. Difficulty listening, careless mistakes, procrastination, easily distracted, forgetful, poor organization, difficulty completing tasks

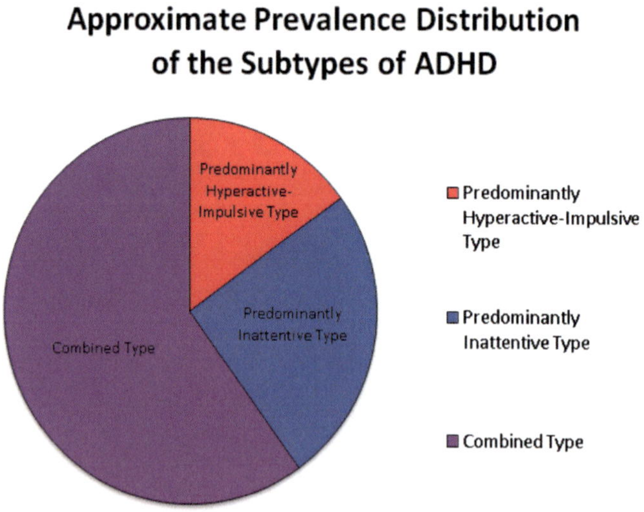

FIGURE 19.1.9 - Approximate Prevalence Distribution of the Different Types of ADHD

IV. ADHD: Diagnosis
   A. Pattern of behavior positive for multiple symptoms in ≥2 settings (hyperactivity/impulsivity and inattention)
   B. Symptoms:
      1. Present for ≥ 6 months
      2. Onset: < age 12
      3. Disproportionate for the developmental stage of the individual
   C. Impaired functionality (social, academic, emotional)

V. ADHD: Adults
   A. The diagnostic criteria for children and adults are similar
   B. Some hyperactive and impulsive symptoms diminish with age
   C. Inattentive symptoms usually persist
      1. Problems at work: goal creation, organization, task completion
   D. Symptoms present since childhood (prior to age 12)
   E. Increased risk of mood disorders and substance abuse

VI. ADHD: Comorbidities
   A. Tourette syndrome
   B. Mood disorders
   C. Behavioral disorders
   D. Specific learning disorder

VII. ADHD: Treatment
   A. Stimulants (methylphenidate)
   B. α_2-adrenergic-agonists (atomoxetine, clonidine, guanfacine)
   C. CBT

VIII. Specific Learning Disorder
   A. Inability to understand a specific subject despite >6 months of help
   B. Diagnosis
      1. Normal intelligence and functionality
      2. Poor learning ability in one subject; low test scores
      3. Educational testing, hearing/vision screening, psychiatric illness
   C. Comorbidities: autism, ADHD, behavioral disorders
   D. Treatment: counseling, tutoring, after school activities

IX. Intellectual Disability
   A. Global deficits of intellectual functioning (e.g. problem solving, general learning ability) and adaptive skills (e.g. reading, social communication, bathing)
   B. Diagnosis
      1. Deficits in BOTH intellectual and adaptive functioning
      2. Daily functional impairment in a variety of settings
   C. Treatment: multidisciplinary support (family support, special education, life skill development)

X. Autism Spectrum Disorder
   A. Deficits in social interaction and restricted interests/behaviors
      1. 4x more common in boys; larger head and brain size
   B. Diagnosis
      1. Symptoms present during early childhood
      2. Social deficits
      3. Insistence on routines
      4. Altered sensory perception
      5. Restricted, repetitive, and ritualistic patterns of behavior

XI. Autism Spectrum Disorder: Savants
   A. Savant: detailed knowledge in a specific field
   B. Example:
      1. An autistic adolescent that knows everything about quantum mechanics
   C. Rare among those with autism

XII. Autism Spectrum Disorder: Treatment
   A. Educational and behavioral therapy
   B. Early diagnosis is key

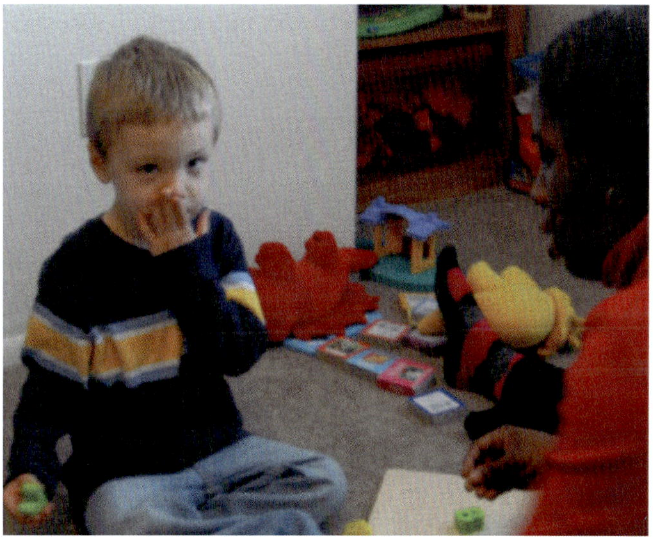

Photo Credit: https://www.edwards.af.mil/News/Photos/igphoto/2000295349/

FIGURE 19.1.10 - Child with Autism Spectrum Disorder

REVIEW QUESTIONS

1. A 24-year-old male began working at a new job 4 months ago but was recently told that he needs to make some changes or else he will be fired. His boss is concerned because he is constantly interrupting others, frequently fidgets, and has spent company funds on useless items without proper permission. This type of behavior has been apparent since the patient was 16-years-old. Does he have ADHD?

    - **No, this patient does not have ADHD.**
    - This patient has some hyperactive symptoms that could potentially indicate ADHD - he interrupts others, frequently fidgets, and has some impulsive behaviors such as spending company funds on useless items without proper permission.
    - However, there are two key points that make ADHD unlikely - first there was no mention of these symptoms occurring in two settings - only work was mentioned.
    - And second, this type of behavior has only been apparent since he was 16-years-old.
    - In order to diagnoseADHD in an adult, symptoms of inattention, hyperactivity, and impulsivity must have been present since before the age of 12.
    - Therefore, this individual does not meet the diagnostic criteria for ADHD.

2. A 4-year-old male recently began attending daycare while his parents work. His teachers have noted some odd behaviors especially when it comes to interacting with other children. He enjoys playing alone with his train toys. When other children try to play and move the trains out of order, he becomes upset and has emotional outbursts. He also becomes incredibly agitated when he hears the sirens passing from the firehouse nearby. Based on this patient's actions what is the most likely diagnosis?

    A. Attention-deficit hyperactivity disorder
    B. Conduct disorder
    C. Oppositional defiant disorder
    D. Normal childhood behavior
    E. Specific learning disorder

    - **The correct answer is A.**
    - The key points for ADHD include difficulties in school, history of forgetting things easily, procrastination, constant fidgeting and playing with his clothes during the interview. The behavior is causing problems in school and is abnormal for his stage of development.
    - He doesn't demonstrate the cruel acts associated with conduct disorder, so B is incorrect.
    - He does have a bad attitude about school, but he doesn't seem to be openly defiant or vindictive like children with oppositional defiant disorder, so C is incorrect.
    - While aspects of his behavior may be normal for an adolescent, collectively they are abnormal and are consistent with a diagnosis of ADHD so D is incorrect.
    - He also isn't struggling with one subject in particular like what we'd see in specific learning disorder, so E is incorrect.

Psychiatry | Section 4: Depression

I. Mood
   A. An emotional state
   B. Extreme sadness → depression
   C. Extreme happiness → mania

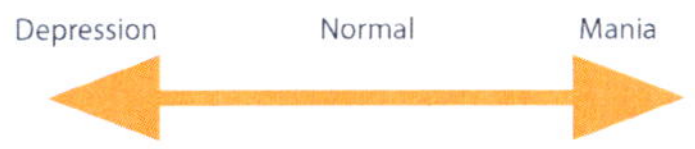

II. SIG E CAPS
   A. Sleep disturbances: hypersomnia or insomnia
   B. Interests: loss of interest in most (or all) activities
   C. Guilt: thoughts of worthlessness or inappropriate guilt
   D. Energy: fatigue or decreased energy
   E. Concentration: inability to focus or make decisions
   F. Appetite/weight: appetite and significant weight changes
   G. Psychomotor: agitation or retardation
   H. Suicidal ideation: recurrent thoughts of death or suicide

III. Suicide Risk Factors
   A. Mnemonic: SAD PERSONS WEEP
      1. Sex (women attempt and men complete)
      2. Age (young or elderly)
      3. Depression
      4. Prior attempt (strongest risk factor)
      5. Ethanol (drugs)
      6. Rational loss of thinking (psychosis)
      7. Sickness (medical illness)
      8. Organized plan
      9. No social support or spouse
      10. Stated intent
      11. Weapons (firearms)
      12. Employment loss
      13. Exemplified by family
      14. Psychiatric hospitalization

IV. MDD: Treatment
   A. Antidepressant trial (e.g. fluoxetine): 4-6 weeks
   B. If this fails, physician may consider:
      1. Adding psychotherapy
      2. Switching to another antidepressant (e.g. bupropion, venlafaxine)
      3. Adding another antidepressant
   C. Continuation phase treatment:
      1. Continuing treatment for six months after initial remission
      2. For patients with single episode
   D. Maintenance phase treatment:
      1. 1-2 years: ≥ 2 episodes, residual depressive symptoms
      2. Lifelong treatment: ≥ 3 episodes, chronic episodes (≥ 2 years), severe features (e.g. suicide attempt)

V. Serotonin Syndrome
   A. Causes:
      1. Overdose or combination of serotonergic drugs (e.g. SSRIs, SNRIs, TCAs, tramadol, meperidine, phenelzine, linezolid)
   B. Clinical features, classic triad of:
      1. Altered mental status (e.g. delirium, agitation, confusion)
      2. Neuromuscular excitability (e.g. hyperreflexia, clonus, tremor)
      3. Autonomic disturbances (e.g. hyperthermia, hypertension, tachycardia, nausea, vomiting)
   C. Management:
      1. Discontinue the implicated drug
      2. Supportive measures (e.g. hydration, cold compresses, antihypertensives, benzodiazepines)
      3. Cyproheptadine (serotonin receptor antagonist)

VI. Electroconvulsive Therapy
   A. Electrodes are used to induce a seizure under general anesthesia
   B. Uses
      1. Severe (treatment resistant) depression
      2. Bipolar disorder; MDD with psychotic symptoms
      3. Schizophrenia/schizoaffective disorder
      4. Acute suicidality
   C. Safety and efficacy: no contraindications
   D. Side effects: headache, disorientation, amnesia; resolve <6 months

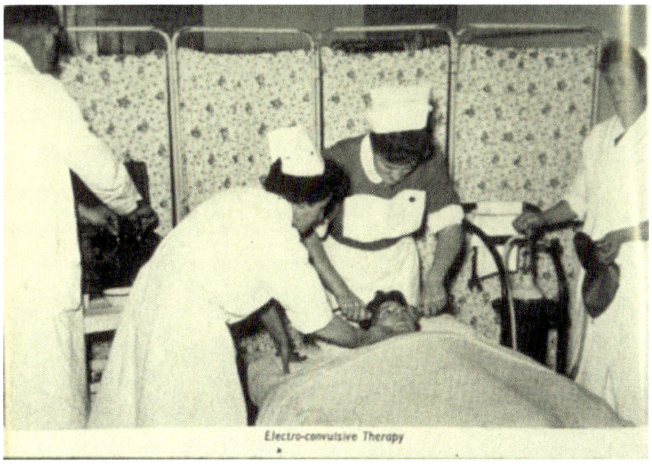

Photo Credit: University of Liverpool Faculty of Health & Life Sciences [Flickr]

FIGURE 19.1.11 - Electroconvulsive Therapy

VII. Clinical Presentations Similar to Depression
   A. Normal sadness
   B. Grief
   C. Complicated grief

VIII. Normal Sadness
  A. Depressed mood
  B. Less than 5 SIG E CAPS symptoms
  C. No functional impairment
  D. Treatment unnecessary

IX. Grief
  A. Normal response that is usually due to the loss of a loved one
  B. Shares symptoms with MDD (e.g. sadness, insomnia, poor appetite, weight loss)
  C. May have > 5 SIG E CAPS (concurrent MDD)
  D. Thoughts of dying are centered on a yearning to be with the deceased
  E. Reduction in symptom severity within 6-12 months of bereavement
  F. 5-stages ("losing a loved one feels BAADD"): bargaining, anger, acceptance, denial, & depression

X. Complicated Grief
  A. Similar to typical grief but with more severe symptoms
    1. Persistent yearning for the deceased
    2. Frequent thoughts about the person who died
    3. Intense urge to join the decreased
    4. Depressive symptoms
    5. Symptoms persist > 6 months
    6. Functional impairment

Disease	Time	Key Features	Other	Treatment
Major depressive disorder (MDD)	≥ 2 consecutive weeks	- At least one episode of ≥5 diagnostic symptoms for ≥2 weeks (self-reported depressed mood or anhedonia required)	- SIG E CAPS	- 1st line: CBT & SSRIs - 2nd line: bupropion, mirtazapine, & SNRIs - Other: ECT for treatment resistant patients
MDD with psychotic features	≥ 2 consecutive weeks	- Major depressive episode that simultaneously occurs with psychotic features (e.g. hallucinations, delusions, disorganized thought)		- Antidepressants and antipsychotics or ECT
Persistent depressive disorder (dysthymia)	≥ 2 years	- ≥ 2 depressive symptoms lasting ≥ 2 years - Will have periods of a normal mood but these cannot last longer than 2 months	- 2 sad for 2 long	- CBT ± antidepressants
MDD with seasonal pattern	≥ 2 years	- ≥ 2 MDD episodes associated with a seasonal pattern (usually late Fall or Winter) - Associated with atypical symptoms (e.g. leaden paralysis, hyperphagia, hypersomnia)		- CBT, antidepressants, & light therapy (winter)
Depression with atypical features		- Mood reactivity (mostly depression but some improvement with positive events) - Rejection sensitivity - Associated with atypical symptoms (e.g. leaden paralysis, hyperphagia, hypersomnia)	- Most common subtype of depression	- 1st line: CBT & SSRIs - MAO inhibitors less often (dangerous side effects)
Maternal (postpartum) blues	Begins 2-3 days postpartum and resolves by day 10	- Overwhelming fatigue, sadness, insomnia, brain fog, & daily functioning difficulties; suicidal ideation should not be present	- Incidence of 50-85%	- Supportive + follow-up
MDD with peripartum onset	Begins within the 1st month postpartum and lasts ≥ 2 weeks	- Meets criteria for major depressive episode after giving birth - Suicidal ideation can be present	- Incidence of 10-15%	- CBT - SSRIs
Postpartum psychosis	Begins within 2 weeks postpartum	- Hallucinations, delusions, homicidal/ suicidal thoughts - Risk factors include discontinuing medication, a history of bipolar or psychotic disorders, family history, and first pregnancy	- Incidence of 0.1-0.2%	- Hospitalization - Antipsychotics - ECT

TABLE 19.1.4 - Depressive Disorders

REVIEW QUESTIONS

1. A 45-year-old woman is brought to the emergency department due to confusion for the past 4 hours. She has been taking fluoxetine for major depressive disorder for 2 years. She was also prescribed linezolid for cellulitis of her foot 1 week ago. Her vital signs include a temperature of 40 C (104 F), a blood pressure of 180/100 mmHg, a heart rate of 125 beats/min, and a respiratory rate of 25 breaths/min. The physical examination reveals 4+ reflexes diffusely along with clonus. In addition to supportive measures, which medication is likely to reverse this patient's current condition?

    - **In addition to supportive measures such as cold compresses, antihypertensives, and benzodiazepines, this patient is likely to benefit from cyproheptadine. Cyproheptadine is serotonin receptor antagonist with antihistamine effects and is likely to alleviate symptoms of serotonin syndrome.**
    - This woman is brought due to acute confusion.
    - She has been taking fluoxetine, an SSRI, for major depressive disorder for 2 years.
    - She was also prescribed linezolid for cellulitis of her foot 1 week ago.
    - Linezolid has partial inhibitory effect on monoamine oxidase so it increases serotonin levels in central nervous system.
    - Combination of linezolid with SSRI likely triggered serotonin syndrome in this patient.
    - Serotonin syndrome is further supported by signs of autonomic instability such as hyperthermia with the temperature of 40 C, high blood pressure of 180/100 mmHg, and tachycardia with the heart rate of 125 beats/min,
    - The physical examination reveals 4+ reflexes diffusely along with clonus which further support the diagnosis of serotonin syndrome.

2. A 43-year-old woman presents to her physician due to insomnia. She states that she went through a divorce three weeks ago and has felt depressed since the event. She also finds herself feeling guilty about putting her children through this experience. She denies weight gain, fatigue, or suicidal ideation. She also continues to enjoy spending time with friends and reading books. Physical examination is normal. Laboratory results show a TSH level of 2.5 µU/mL (normal: 0.5-5.0 µU/mL) and a free T4 of 7 µU/dL (normal: 5-12 µU/dL). What is the most likely diagnosis?

    A. Normal sadness
    B. Grief
    C. Complicated grief
    D. Hypothyroidism
    E. Major depressive disorder

    - **The correct answer is A.**
    - From the question stem we can see that this patient went through a divorce and is now experiencing some depressive symptoms.
    - She has insomnia, has felt depressed, and has had difficulting concentrating for three weeks.
    - It's important to note that she still enjoys hobbies in her life and isn't suicidal so this is normal sadness and the correct answer is A.
    - B and C are incorrect because the question stem says nothing about the loss of a loved one.
    - D is incorrect because her TSH And free T4 levels are normal.
    - Finally E is incorrect because she only has 3 of the SIG E CAPS symptoms.
    - Remember, 5 SIG E CAPS symptoms for two weeks is required to diagnose MDD.

REVIEW QUESTIONS ?

3. A 33-year-old female presents to the office due to a prolonged feeling of sadness. She says she first noticed this feeling approximately 3 years ago. She also mentions that she always feels guilty about mistakes made from her past. She endorses periods of feeling happy, but these are typically short lived and only last a few weeks at a time. What is the most likely diagnosis?

- **The most likely diagnosis of this patient is dysthymia.**
- This patient has felt sad (sadness) and guilty for 3 years.
- She has also had periods of feeling happy but these only last a few weeks.
- From the table, recall that dysthymia is characterized by two or more MDD symptoms the last for 2 or more years and that patients can have periods of a normal mood but that these cannot last longer than 2 months.
- This is perfectly describing the patient from the question.

4. A 43-year-old woman comes to the office for a yearly checkup. She states that her daughter passed away in a car accident five months ago and is very sad about the incident. She has difficulty leaving the house, feels intense anger toward the person who hit her daughter with their car, cries often, and regularly thinks about her daughter longingly. At the end of the interview she smiles as she shares what she loved most about her daughter. Which of the following is the most likely diagnosis?

F. Complicated grief
G. Grief
H. Major depressive disorder
I. Normal sadness
J. Dysthymia
K. Depression with atypical features

- **The correct answer is B.**
- This woman lost her daughter five months ago and is now experiencing some sadness.
- She has difficulty leaving the house, feels intense anger, cries, and thinks about her daughter regularly.
- Remember, if a question mentions the loss of a loved one then you should immediately begin thinking about grief.
- A is wrong because her symptoms haven't lasted longer than 6 months and they aren't so severe that they're causing functional impairment or depression.
- C is wrong because she only has a depressed mood and possibly some anhedonia because she has difficulty leaving the house.
- However, 2 out of 5 of the SIG E CAPS symptoms is not sufficient to make this diagnosis.
- D is wrong because the question stem states that she lost her daughter and these symptoms have been going on for over 5 months.
- Normal sadness would not cause any functional impairment and is unlikely in the setting of recently losing a loved one.
- E is wrong because this patient has only had symptoms for 5 months - not 2 years.
- F is wrong because this patient doesn't have rejection sensitivity or leaden paralysis and she just lost a loved one so grief fits better with this picture.

Psychiatry | Section 5: Mania

I. Mood
   A. An emotional state
   B. Extreme sadness → depression
   C. Extreme happiness → mania

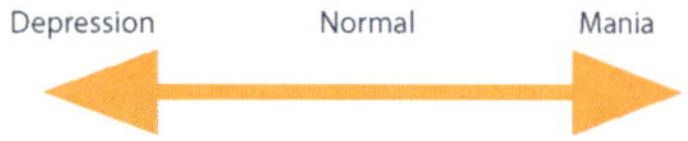

II. DIG FAST
   A. Distractibility
   B. Impulsivity/indiscretion (decisions, sexual impulsivity, spending)
   C. Grandiosity/goals
   D. Flight of ideas: unable to focus
   E. Agitation/activity (restless behavior, goal-directed hyperactivity)
   F. Sleep reduced
   G. Talkative (pressured speech)

III. Treatment
   A. Mild/moderate manic episode or hypomanic episode:
   B. Risperidone or olanzapine
   C. Severe manic episode:
      1. Lithium + antipsychotic (e.g. haloperidol, quetiapine, olanzapine)
      2. Alternative: valproate + antipsychotic
      3. Electroconvulsive therapy may be considered
   D. Hospitalization for severe and suicidal cases
   E. Maintenance therapy:
      1. Start with monotherapy: lithium, valproate, quetiapine, lamotrigine
      2. If unresponsive: lithium or valproate + SGA (e.g. quetiapine)
      3. Avoid lithium in renal diseases and valproate in liver diseases
   F. Usually given for years but in some conditions like suicidal attempts, frequent episodes and hospitalization, lifelong therapy is required

IV. Lithium Toxicity
   A. Narrow therapeutic index
   B. Medications can precipitate lithium toxicity: thiazide diuretics, NSAIDs, ACE inhibitors
   C. Clinical features of lithium toxicity:
      1. Nausea, vomiting, diarrhea
      2. Confusion, encephalopathy, delirium, seizures, coma
      3. Tremors, fasciculations, ataxia, nystagmus
   D. Long-term adverse effects:
      1. Nephrogenic diabetes insipidus
      2. Hypothyroidism; hyperparathyroidism
      3. Chronic kidney disease
   E. Management:
      1. Stop using lithium and/or precipitating medications
      2. Hydration and electrolyte correction to facilitate lithium clearance
      3. Consider hemodialysis in severe toxicity
      4. Beta blockers for tremor and amiloride for nephrogenic DI

Disease	Time	Key Features	Other	Memory Hook
Manic episode	> 1 week or hospital admission	- Persistently elevated, expansive, or irritable mood and abnormally increased energy/activity - May include psychotic features - Diagnosis requires functional impairment with ≥3 manic symptoms	- Mood stabilizers - Antipsychotics	DIG FAST
Hypomanic episodes	≥ 4 days	- Same symptoms as a manic episode without psychotic features - Distinct because there is no functional impairment	- Mood stabilizers - Antipsychotics	
Bipolar I	≥ 1 manic episode	- At least one manic episode ± hypomanic or depressive episode	- Mood stabilizers - Antipsychotics - Avoid antidepressants (destabilize mood)	Mania = 1
Bipolar II	≥ 1 hypomanic and depressive episode	- Both hypomanic and depressive episodes with no history of a manic episode - Mood may stabilize between episodes - High suicide risk	- Mood stabilizers - Antipsychotics - Avoid antidepressants (destabilize mood)	Hypomania + depression = 2
Cyclothymic disorder	≥ 2 years	- Milder form of bipolar disease - Fluctuate between mild depressive symptoms and hypomanic symptoms - Symptoms for ≥ 2 years, present > ½ the time, with remission lasting no longer than 2 months	- Mood stabilizers - Antipsychotics - Avoid antidepressants (destabilize mood)	

TABLE 19.1.5 - Manic-Related Mood Disorders

REVIEW QUESTIONS

1. A 26-year-old male presents to the clinic at his girlfriend's request. For the last 4 days he reports high levels of energy and decreased need for sleep. He states he feels happy and is excited to have been getting so much work done over the past few days. He works from 6 am to 4 pm as a financial analyst then comes home and works until 2 am on a new business proposal. He denies any hallucinations or delusions. What is this patient's most likely diagnosis?
   - **Based on the length of symptoms, 4 days, and the absence of psychotic symptoms and impaired functionality, this patient is most likely suffering from a hypomanic episode**
   - For the last 4 days, this patient reports high levels of energy and decreased need for sleep.
   - His mood is happy and excited.
   - He is working from 6 am until 2 am daily between his day job and writing a new business proposal.
   - He does not have any hallucinations or delusions.
   - This patient has similar symptoms of manic episode such as elevated mood with increased energy.
   - However, he does not have any psychotic features such as hallucinations or delusions.
   - Also, he does not experience functional impairment.

2. A 34-year-old female presents to the office due to persistent feelings of decreased mood. She states she has felt this way for most days over the past 3 years. However, she states that about once every month or two she has two to three days of increased mood and energy. She always thinks this means she is getting better but then always starts to feel down again. She has no symptoms of anhedonia, suicidality, hallucinations, or delusions. What is the treatment for her most likely diagnosis?
   - **The treatment for her most likely diagnosis of clycothymic disorder is mood stabilizers and antipsychotics.**
   - This patient has persistent feelings of decreased mood for most days over the past 3 years.
   - About once a month or so she has 2 or 3 days of increased mood and energy.
   - Since her only depressive symptom is decreased mood and she does not have any further depressive symptoms such as anhedonia or suicidality, she does not meet criteria for major depressive disorder.
   - Also since her only manic symptoms are increased mood & energy lasting less than 4 days and she does not have psychotic symptoms of hallucinations or delusions she does not meet criteria for mania or hypomania.
   - Due to these symptoms persisting for over 2 years (3 years), she most likely has cyclothymic disorder.
   - Cyclothymic disorder can be treated with mood stabilizers and antipsychotics.
   - Remember, do not treat any bipolar or bipolar-associated disorders with antidepressants due to the potential for increasing manic mood symptoms.

REVIEW QUESTIONS

1. A 21-year-old female presents to the clinic with her mother. While she was home from college her mother noticed that she wasn't sleeping. She mentions that for the past 2 weeks the patient has had minimal sleep and has been increasingly energetic. The patient explains that she has only been so energetic because she knows she will bring peace to the world one day and has been planning how. While talking with the patient, she quickly jumps from one idea to the next. Her mother does not know what to do to help the patient who has been ignoring her friends and family since this episode began. What is this patient's most likely diagnosis?

   - **This patient's most likely diagnosis is a manic episode.**
   - This patient presents due to minimal sleep for the past 2 weeks and increased energy.
   - She admits some grandiose plans to bring peace to the world one day.
   - She is also exhibiting flight of ideas.
   - This recent episode is also clearly impairing the patient's daily life.
   - Based on this presentation the patient is having a manic episode.
   - The treatment for this acute episode depends on its severity but generally includes mood stabilizers, such as lithium or valproate, and/or antipsychotics.

2. A 42-year-old male with a history of bipolar I disorder presents to the clinic complaining of drinking water and urinating all the time. He states it has been progressing for the last few months to the point where he is waking up at night 3-4 times to urinate. A quick urinalysis in office shows that his urine osmolality is 180 mOsm/kg water (NL: 500-800 mOsm/kg water). Vital signs are heart rate of 70 beats/min, respiratory rate of 16 breaths/min, blood pressure of 125/80 mmHg, temperature of 99.1°F, and O2 saturation of 99%. The physical examination shows dry mucous membranes. Based on this patient's presentation, what is the most likely cause of his current condition?

   A. Dehydration
   B. Olanzapine toxicity
   C. Lithium toxicity
   D. Ingestion of vasopressin

   - **The correct answer is C.**
   - This patient with a history of bipolar I disorder presents due to drinking water and urinating all the time.
   - He also has symptoms of nocturia by waking up at night to urinate 3-4 times.
   - A urinalysis shows significantly low urine osmolality, meaning that his urine is very dilute.
   - Physical examination shows dry mucous membranes.
   - Based on this patient's excessive thirst, increased urination, and low urine osmolality he most likely has diabetes insipidus.
   - Due to this patient's history of bipolar disorder, answer choice C is the correct answer.
   - This is because lithium is known to cause nephrogenic diabetes insipidus, in the clinic you could determine whether the diabetes insipidus was nephrogenic or central by giving the patient exogenous ADH, aka vasopressin.
   - In central DI, the patient's kidneys would respond to vasopressin by retaining water.
   - In nephrogenic DI, the patient's kidneys would not respond to vasopressin and he would continue to lose water through excessive urination.
   - Based on this, answer choice D is incorrect since if a patient ingested vasopressin, they would retain water not lose it.
   - Answer choice A is incorrec, because if the patient were dehydrated the body would release ADH to retain water not lose it.
   - Answer choice B is incorrect, because the side effects of olanzapine include weight gain and excessive sleepiness not DI.

Psychiatry | Section 6: Anxiety Disorders

Disorder	Symptoms	Diagnosis	Treatment/Therapy
Panic disorder	- Panic attack - ≥ 1 of the following: - fearing more attacks - fear of consequences of attacks - behavior change (eg, avoid leaving house, agoraphobia)	≥ 1 month	- CBT, SSRIs, & SNRIs - Acute attack: benzodiazepines
Generalized anxiety disorder	- Excessive worry about daily life, most days - Restlessness, muscle tension, irritability, disruptions in sleep or concentration, fatigue	≥ 3 symptoms for ≥ 6 months	- 1st line: CBT, SSRIs, & SNRIs - 2nd line: buspirone & benzodiazepines
Obsessive-compulsive disorder	- Intrusive thoughts (obsessions) followed by repetitive actions (compulsions) - Egodystonic - Associated with Tourette syndrome - Body dysmorphic disorder: - Obsession: cosmetic imperfection - Compulsion: repetitive mirror-checking, surgeries	Obsessions and compulsions	- 1st line: CBT, SSRIs, & SNRIs - 2nd line: clomipramine
Phobias - agoraphobia	- Fear of extremely open or closed spaces due to inability to flee	≥ 6 months with specific fear in at least 2 situations	- CBT & SSRIs
Phobias - social anxiety disorder	- Extreme fear of social embarrassment	≥ 6 months	- CBT & SSRIs - Performance: β-blockers or benzodiazepines
Phobias - specific phobias	- Exaggerated fear of one specific object or situation (e.g. spiders, heights)	≥ 6 months	- 1st line: CBT and exposure therapy - 2nd line: benzodiazepines
Trichotillomania	- Compulsive pulling out of one's hair - Areas of thin hair, or hair shafts of different lengths		- CBT (pharmacotherapy less useful)

TABLE 19.1.6 - Anxiety Disorders

I. Anxiety Disorders
   A. A group of psychiatric disorders in which a stress response is out of proportion to the stressor

I. Panic Attack
   A. Sudden surge of fear
   B. May or may not have a trigger
   C. Symptoms peak at 10 minutes and slowly subside
   D. Presents with ≥ 4 of the following symptoms:
      1. Palpitations, chest pain, sweating, shaking, shortness of breath, abdominal pain, nausea, lightheaded, paresthesias, derealization, depersonalization, fear of losing control, fear of dying

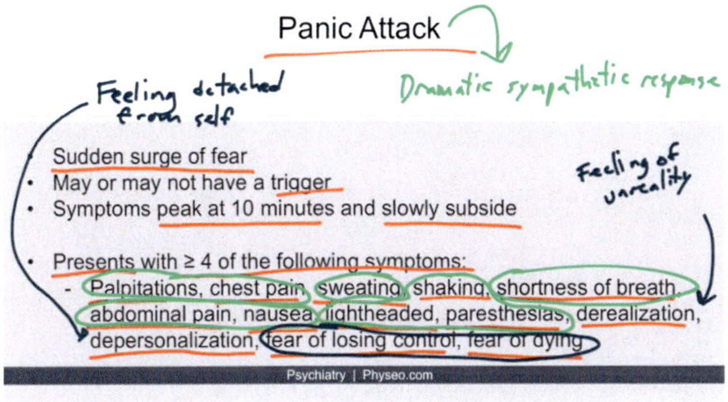

Obsession	Compulsion
safety	lock the front door 12x
sanitation	re-wash hands 6x

II. Exposure Therapy
   A. Gradually increase exposure to the phobia → helps the patient build confidence that the fear is irrational

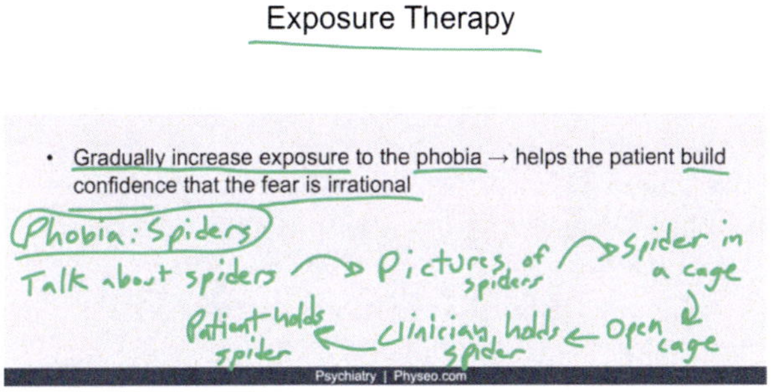

REVIEW QUESTIONS

1. A 23-year-old woman presents to the physician due to fear leaving her house for the past 3 months. She thinks she "is going crazy" and cannot control her emotions. She reports unpredictable episodes of palpitations, sweating, dizziness, and chest pain that typically last for 10-15 minutes. There is no identifiable trigger and the episodes resolve spontaneously. Which class of medications can be used in an acute setting for this patient's underlying condition?

   - **Benzodiazepines is the class of mediciations that can be used for this patient.**
   - This young woman has been afraid of leaving her house for the past 3 months.
   - She reports unpredictable episodes of palpitations, sweating, dizziness, and chest pain that typically last for 10-15 minutes.
   - There is no identifiable trigger and the episodes resolve spontaneously.
   - This description is consistent with the panic episodes.
   - Recurrent panic episodes with disrupted social functioning suggest the diagnosis of panic disorder.
   - Benzodiazepines can be used for sedation in an acute setting in a patient with panic disorder.
   - However, as mentioned on the previous slide, the long-term treatment consists of CBT, SSRIs, or SNRIs.

2. An 8-year-old boy is brought to the physician by his mother who complains of changes in his mood. For the past 8 months, he has been worried about being criticized by his peers in math class and losing his parents. He is also worried about someone breaking into their house and stealing his toys. The mother reports a stable and positive home environment without recent conflicts. The physical examination reveals muscle tension. What is the most likely diagnosis in this patient?

   - **The most likely diagosis in this patient is Generalized Anxiety Disorder or GAD.**
   - This 8-year-old boy has been excessively worried about multiple things for the past 8 months.
   - Additionally, the physical examination reveals muscle tension.
   - These signs and symptoms along with the time frame of more than 6 months are consistent with the diagnosis of generalized anxiety disorder.
   - It is important to note that while three symptoms, in addition to the excessive worry, are needed to diagnose GAD in adults, the presence of even one symptom, muscle tension in our case, for at least 6 months is sufficient to diagnose GAD in children

REVIEW QUESTIONS

3. A 32-year-old woman comes to the physician due to difficulty "controlling her thoughts" for the past 6 months. She commonly thinks about germs on her bed linens and asymmetric roof of her house. Whenever these thoughts come, she starts counting out loud to mitigate the thoughts. She feels distressed and embarrassed by her behavior. What are the first-line treatment options for this patient?

- **The first-line treatment option for this patient for their OCD includes cognitive-helavioral therapy, SSRIs, and SNRIs.**
- This young woman reports difficulty "controlling her thoughts" for the past 6 months.
- She commonly thinks about germs on her bed linens and asymmetric roof of her house.
- These are obsessions, or intrusive, unwanted thoughts.
- Whenever these thoughts come, she starts counting out loud to mitigate the thoughts.
- Counting in this case is an example of compulsion.
- Compulsion is the physical or mental act that at least partially alleviates obsession-induced anxiety.
- Obsessions and compulsions are consistent with the diagnosis of obsessive-compulsive disorder, or OCD.
- The first-line treatment options for OCD include cognitive-behavioral therapy, SSRIs, and SNRIs.

4. A 41-year-old businessman comes to the physician due to severe anxiety for the past 7 months. Everytime he leaves his house for work, he thinks something bad is going to happen on the way and he will not be able to escape. These thoughts make him avoid crowded places. He also reports getting a little "panicky and shaky" before business meetings but he is able to calm down once he starts talking. He is concerned about his finances and relationship with his wife. Vital signs are unremarkable. The physical examination reveals a restless man in no distress. Which of the following is the most likely diagnosis in this patient?

    A. Generalized anxiety disorder
    B. Panic disorder
    C. Agoraphobia
    D. Social anxiety disorder

- **The correct answer is C.**
- This man presents with severe anxiety for the past 7 months.
- Everytime he leaves his house fo job, he thinks something bad is going to happen on the way and he will not be able to escape.
- These thoughts make him avoid crowded places and queues.
- Vital signs are unremarkable and the physical examination reveals a restless man in no distress.
- Avoidance of public spaces due to fear of not being to escape in case something bad happens is consistent with the diagnosis of agoraphobia.
- Therefore, correct answer is option C.
- Option A is incorrect because generalized anxiety disorder requires the presence of at least 3 symptoms for at least 6 months.
- This patient is worried and restless but he does not fully meet the criteria for generalized anxiety disorder.
- Option B is incorrect because the diagnosis of panic disorder requires the presence of panic episodes.
- Although this patient gets a little "panicky and shaky" before business meetings, panic episode needs at least 4 symptoms.
- Finally option D is incorrect because although he feels anxious before meetings, he is able to calm down once he starts talking.
- In contrast, patients with social anxiety disorder have difficulty calming down even after they start the public speech.

Psychiatry | Section 7: Cognition, Orientation, Delirium & Amnesia

I. Cognition
   A. The process of understanding through thought and experience
      1. Language
      2. Memory
      3. Reasoning
      4. Attention
      5. Orientation

II. Neurocognitive Disorders
   A. Amnesia
   B. Delirium
   C. Dementia

III. Amnesia
   A. Retrograde Amnesia
      1. Can make new memories but unable to remember anything prior to CNS insult (befoRE)
   B. Anterograde Amnesia
      1. Can remember everything before the CNS insult but cannot form new memories (After)

IV. Korsakoff Syndrome
   A. Pathophysiology
      1. Alcoholism → thiamine (B1) deficiency → Wernicke encephalopathy (acute) → mamillary body destruction & Korsakoff syndrome (chronic)
   B. Symptoms
      1. Anterograde amnesia (retrograde also possible)
      2. Confabulations (no intent to deceive)

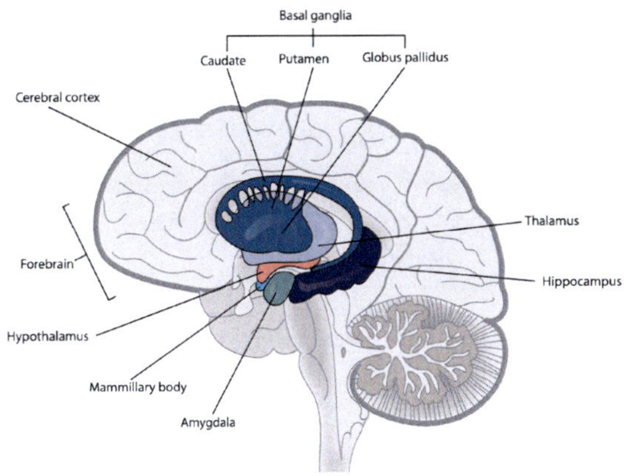

FIGURE 19.1.12 - The Limbic System and Basal Ganglia

V. Delirium
   A. Definition:
      1. Acute (reversible) loss of cognitive function
      2. Waxes and wanes
      3. Hyperactive (agitated) or hypoactive (sluggish)
      4. Psychotic features common (delusions, hallucinations)
   B. Causes (pathophysiology not well understood):
      1. Medications
      2. Infections
      3. Hospital overnight
      4. Trauma or organ dysfunction of any kind
   C. Treatment:
      1. Fix underlying problem
      2. Open the blinds during the day
      3. Antipsychotics (if safety is an issue)

VI. Dementia
   A. Decline in cognitive function
   B. Chronic
   C. Irreversible
   D. Progressive

REVIEW QUESTIONS ?

1. A 73-year-old woman is recovering in a hospital room on day 2 following an abdominal surgery. The physician began asking her questions and found that the patient knew her name, but didn't know the year or the name of the city. The remainder of the interview was difficult because the patient was very slow to respond and needed to be prompted multiple times before a question was answered. What information is required to tell if this patient has dementia or delirium?
   - **This patient has delirium. The information required to diagnose this as delirium is based on cognitive functions including language, memory, reasoning, attention, and orientation.**
   - This patient had problems with two cognitive processes: orientation and attention.
   - Knowing the onset will discriminate between dementia (a chronic condition) or delirium (an acute condition with a recent onset).

Psychiatry | Section 8: Psychosis

I. Psychosis
   A. Conditions that affect the mind that are characterized by a loss of contact with reality
   B. Can occur due to psychiatric illness, medical illness, or substance use
   C. Key difference from dissociation:
      1. Patients experiencing dissociation are in touch with reality
   D. Key features include delusions, hallucinations, and thought disorganization

II. Delusions, Hallucinations, and Thought Disorganization
   A. Delusions: fixed, false beliefs that cannot be corrected by logic and are not consistent with culture and education of the patient
   B. Hallucinations: false sensory perception experienced without real external stimulus (e.g. seeing a person who is not really present)
   C. Thought disorganization: incoherent, tangential, or derailed thoughts

Delusion	Definition	Example
Definition	Belief that someone is in love with the afflicted person	"Leonardo Dicaprio is in love with me"
Example	Fixed, false belief that a person has superior qualities of genius, wealth, or fame	"I'm going to win an Olympic gold medal"
Jealous	Belief that a spouse or partner is being unfaithful with no proof and accompanied by socially unacceptable behavior	"My wife is cheating on me"
Persecutory	Affected person thinks they are being persecuted	"I am being followed"
Somatic	Affected person thinks their body is diseased or altered in some way with change in feeling, sensation, or appearance	"I have bugs crawling all over my body"
Mixed	When a person experiences delusions from multiple categories	"My food is being poisoned and my husband is cheating on me"
Unspecified	Delusion that does not fit in one of the above categories	"You're not the person you claim to be" Capgras syndrome

TABLE 19.1.7 - Types of Delusions

Hallucination	Definition	Association
Auditory	Involves perceiving sound with no auditory stimulus	More common in psychiatric illness than medical illness
Visual	Perception of external visual stimulus when none exists	More common in medical illness than psychiatric illness
Tactile	False perception of touch when no stimulus exists	Common in alcohol withdrawal and stimulant use
Olfactory	Perception of smell when no external stimulus exists	Can occur as an aura in temporal lobe epilepsy and in brain tumors
Gustatory	Perception of taste when no external stimulus exists	Rare, but seen in epilepsy
Hypnagogic	Transitional state from wakefulness to sleep; when a person hears, smells, or sees something just before falling asleep	Occurs when going to sleep and seen in patients with narcolepsy
Hypnopompic	Vivid dreamlike experiences that can seem real and are often frightening	Occurs while waking from sleep and seen in patients with narcolepsy

TABLE 19.1.8 - Types of Hallucinations

III. Illusions
   A. Misperception of a real external stimulus
   B. Most likely to occur when general level of sensory stimulation (consciousness) is reduced
   C. Can be auditory, visual, or sensory
   D. Not a feature of psychosis

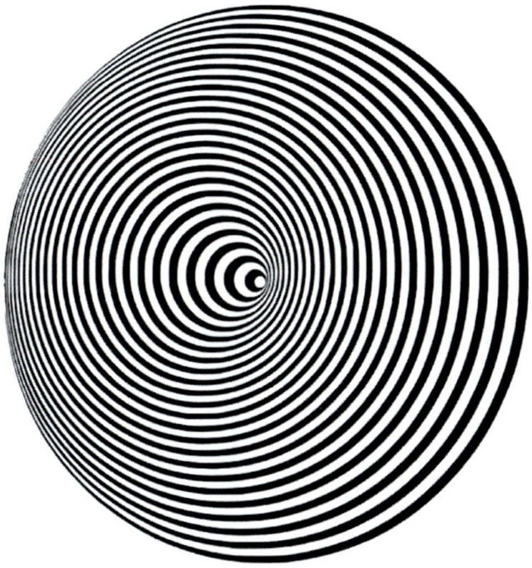

Photo Credit: Creative Common Public Domain

FIGURE 19.1.13 - Optical Illusion

IV. Disorganized Thought
   A. Normal thought process should be linear, goal-directed, and oriented
      1. abnormalities occur in connectivity, speed, or amount of thought
   B. Disorganized thinking is evidenced by disordered speech
      1. may be incoherent, tangential, or derailed

Tangential

"The city of London is in England. I know this from my school days. Then, I always like geography. My last teacher in that subject was professor August A. He was a man with black eyes. I also like black eyes. There are blue and gray eyes and other sorts, too. I have heard it said that snakes have green eyes. All people have eyes, there are some, too, that are blind."

-- Unidentified patient in letter to his mother (Bleuler, 1911)

FIGURE 19.1.14 - Example of Tangential

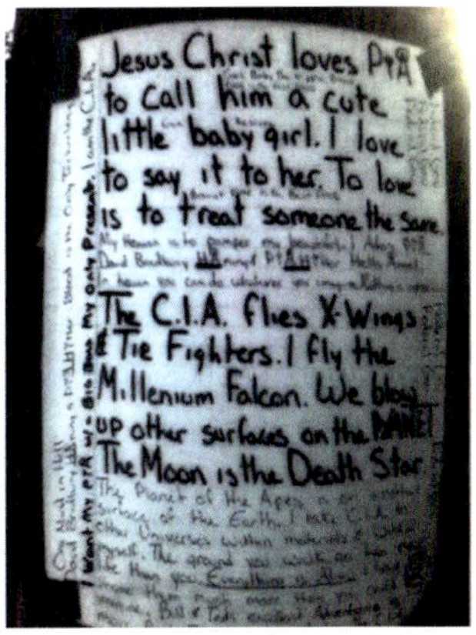

Photo Credit: Photo by mattymatt from Creative Commons

FIGURE 19.1.15 - Loose Associations

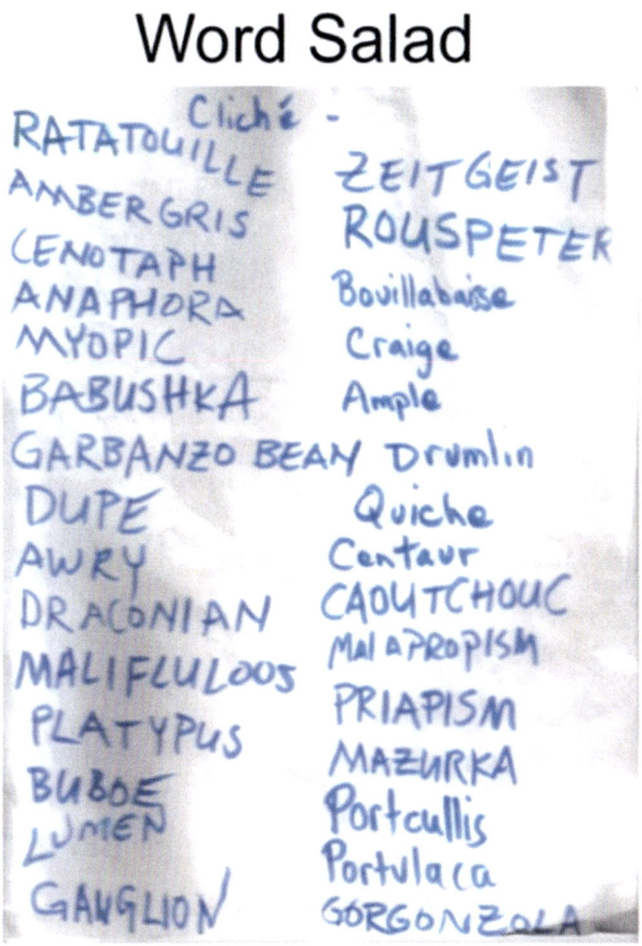

FIGURE 19.1.16 - Word Salad

Clang Associations

You're solar, bipolar
Panic disorder

Systematic, sympathetic
Quite pathetic, apologetic, paramedic
Your heart is prosthetic

FIGURE 19.1.17 - Example of Clang Associations

REVIEW QUESTIONS

1. A 33-year-old male reports seeing someone walk by the hallway while the physician was speaking with him. However, the physician was looking in the same direction and didn't see anyone. Is this normal or evidence of psychosis? Why?

- **The patients behavior is evidence of psychosis.**
- The key feature here is that the patient reported seeing someone but the physician was looking in the same direction and didn't see anything. In other words, there was no external stimulus that caused the patient to see this, so it was a hallucination.
- This is evidence of psychosis because delusions, hallucinations, and thought disorganization are all features of psychosis.
- If the physician saw the light turn on in the hallway while the patient reported seeing someone then this could have been interpreted as an illusion because the external stimulus could have been misinterpreted by the patient.
- However, there was no suggestion that an external stimulus was present so this patient was most likely hallucinating.

2. A 69-year old homeless man presents to the emergency department in obvious distress. He is having a hard time walking in a straight line and when he approaches the desk to check in, he says that he needs protection because he is being "followed" and he continually repeats "they are after me." He tells the doctor not to worry about how he is going to pay for healthcare because he is a millionaire. What type of psychosis is this patient experiencing?

   A. Illusions
   B. Hallucinations
   C. Grandiose delusion
   D. Persecutory delusion
   E. Mixed delusion

- **The correct answer is E.**
- His belief that he is being followed and that someone is after him should make you think of a persecutory delusion. His belief that he is a millionaire is a grandiose delusion.The combination of these two delusions should lead you answer E.
- Illusions is incorrect because there is no external stimulus that creating his feeling of being followed
- Hallucinations is incorrect because he is experiencing symptoms that are more similar to a delusion rather than a hallucination. He does not report any visual, auditory, or somatic hallucinations and is more paranoid than hallucinating
- C and D are both partially correct answers. The patient is experiencing both grandiose and persecutory delusions and therefore those answers are incorrect on their own, but are both parts of a mixed delusion.

Psychiatry | Section 9: Psychotic Disorders

Type	Definition	Timing of Diagnosis	Clinical Presentation
Schizophrenia	Psychiatric disorder involving chronic or recurrent psychosis that causes profound functional impairment	Onset of symptoms > 6 months prior to diagnosis with > 1 month of active symptoms	Hallucinations, delusions, unusual thought process, disorganized speech, etc.
Schizophreniform disorder	All criteria for schizophrenia are met, but total duration of disorder is 1-6 months	1-6 months of active symptoms of schizophrenia	Hallucinations, delusions, unusual thought process, disorganized speech, etc.
Brief psychotic disorder	Presence of one or more psychotic symptoms with a sudden onset and full remission within one month	< 1 month of positive active symptoms	Hallucinations, delusions, disorganized speech, disorganized behavior
Schizoaffective disorder	Schizophrenia with manic episodes or a significant depressive component; psychosis can and does occur in the absence of mood episodes	> 2 weeks of psychotic symptoms without a manic or depressive episode	Symptoms of schizophrenia plus manic episode (high energy, reduced need for sleep, euphoria), or a depressive episode (low energy, low motivation)
Delusional disorder	Disorder involving one or more delusions lasting for over one month, but person is otherwise not functionally impaired	> 1 delusion lasting > 1 month, no other mood disorder or other psychotic symptoms	Symptoms are organized around a delusional concern or theme; can be shared by individuals in close relationships
Schizotypal personality disorder	Chronic personality disorder that manifests in childhood and adolescence; on the schizophrenia spectrum	Cluster A personality disorder; odd or eccentric with no psychotic symptoms	Cognitive perceptual problems, odd rapport, affect, and speech, interpersonal problems

TABLE 19.1.9 - Psychotic Disorders

I. Schizophrenia Symptoms
   A. Positive
      1. Hallucinations, delusions, disorganized thoughts and behavior
   B. Negative
      1. Absence or diminution of normal behavior (eg, flat/blunted affect, apathy, lack of energy, social withdrawal)
   C. Cognitive
      1. Diminished memory, attention span, processing speed

II. Risk Factors
   A. Urban areas
   B. Immigration
   C. Frequent cannabis use
   D. Presents earlier in men than women
      1. Men = 18-25
      2. Women = 25-35
   E. ↑ suicide risk

III. Pathology
   A. ↑ dopamine
   B. ↓ dendritic spines
   C. Ventriculomegaly on brain imaging or autopsy

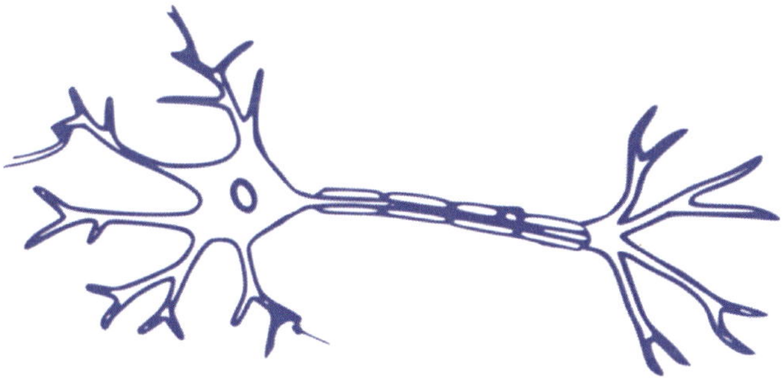

FIGURE 19.1.18 - Dendritic Spines

IV. Schizophrenia Diagnosis
   A. Diagnosis: ≥ 2 active symptoms for ≥ 1 month
      1. Onset: > 6 months prior to diagnosis
      2. Must cause social/occupational dysfunction
   B. Active symptoms:
      1. Delusions*
      2. Hallucinations*
      3. Disorganized speech*
      4. *must have at least one of these three*
   C. Disorganized or catatonic behavior
   D. Negative symptoms

V. Schizoaffective Disorder
   A. Schizophrenia with mood disorder symptoms (significant depression or manic episodes)
   B. Psychosis occurs with AND without mood disorder symptoms
   C. Must be able to distinguish this from a mood disorder with psychotic features
   D. An episode of psychotic symptoms must have occurred for > 2 weeks WITHOUT mood disorder symptoms

VI. Delusional Disorder
   A. Example:
      1. Man thinks his food is poisoned when he eats outside of his house
      2. He makes someone test his food every time he eats
      3. He cannot be convinced his food is safe
      4. No hallucinations, disorganized thought, or negative symptoms

REVIEW QUESTIONS

1. A 21-year-old male is brought to the hospital by his family due to "strange behavior." For the past two months he has been isolated in his apartment because "he's hiding from the aliens." Upon further inquiry he reports multiple encounters with aliens and says that he saw one of them following him in the hall earlier today. Does this patient have schizophrenia?

   - **This patient does not have schizophrenia.**
   - This patient is having delusions because he believes aliens are after him, which is why he's hiding from the aliens. This is a fixed false belief or a delusion.
   - He has also been hallucinating because he reports multiple encounters with aliens and says that he saw one of them. However, the timeline is key here - he has only been having these episodes for the past two months.
   - This means regardless of his delusions and hallucinations, he does not meet the diagnostic criteria for schizophrenia because the symptoms have to be present for at least 6 months. He's only had them for 2 months.

2. A 21-year-old male is brought to the hospital by his family due to "strange behavior." For the past two months he has been isolated in his apartment because "he's hiding from the aliens." Upon further inquiry he reports multiple encounters with aliens and says that he saw one of them following him in the hall earlier today. What is the most likely diagnosis?

   - **The correct answer is schizophreniform disorder.**
   - This patient has had symptoms for two months so this is too long of a timeline to fit with brief psychotic disorder yet too short of a timeline to fit with schizophrenia.
   - The timeline here is super important for distinguishing the different psychotic disorders.

3. A 29-year-old male is brought to the hospital by his wife because he is having a manic episode. He is also hallucinating and delusional. Can this patient be diagnosed with schizoaffective disorder?

   - **No he cannot - this example is describing a mood disorder with psychotic features.**
   - The manic episode is the mood disorder. The hallucinations and delusions just mean that he is also experiencing psychotic features.
   - In other words, this would be diagnosed as a mood disorder with psychotic features.
   - The question says nothing about a prior isolated episode of psychosis so we cannot say that this patient has schizoaffective disorder.

4. A 29-year-old male is brought to the hospital by his wife because he is having a manic episode. He is also hallucinating and delusional. Can this patient be diagnosed with schizoaffective disorder?

   - **No, this example is describing a mood disorder with psychotic features.**
   - So the manic episode is the mood disorder and the hallucinations and delusions just mean that he is also experiencing psychotic features.
   - In other words, this would be diagnosed as a mood disorder with psychotic features.
   - The question says nothing about a prior isolated episode of psychosis so we cannot say that this patient has schizoaffective disorder.

REVIEW QUESTIONS

5. A 29-year-old male is brought to the hospital by his wife because he is having a manic episode. He is also hallucinating and delusional. In the past he has had several episodes lasting several months involving hallucinations and delusions in the absence of mania. Can this patient be diagnosed with schizoaffective disorder?

   - **Yes, this patient a diagnosis of schizoaffective disorder.**
   - The question is slightly different this time because in this example the patient has had several episodes lasting several months involving hallucinations and delusions in the absence of mania.
   - In other words, he was psychotic without any mood disorder symptoms.
   - His acute presentation could be confused with a mood disorder because is manic.
   - However, the prior history really tells us that he has schizoaffective disorder because he had an isolated episode of psychosis that was longer than two weeks.

6. A 24-year-old man is evaluated at the hospital for painful cramps of neck muscles. He has a past medical history of poorly controlled schizophrenia. He was admitted 3 days ago with psychosis and aggressive behavior for which he necessitated several injections of haloperidol. The physical examination reveals a right-sided head tilt with severe spasm of right sternocleidomastoid muscle. Which medications can be used to treat this patient's current condition?

   - **This patient's current condition can be treated with benztropine or diphenhydramine.**
   - This young man is evaluated for painful cramps of neck muscles.
   - He has a past medical history of poorly controlled schizophrenia.
   - He was admitted 3 days ago with psychosis and aggressive behavior for which he necessitated several injections of haloperidol.
   - Haloperidol is a high-potency first-generation antipsychotic with high probability of causing extrapyramidal symptoms.
   - The physical examination reveals a right-sided head tilt with severe spasm of right sternocleidomastoid muscle.
   - This is a classic description of torticollis which, in this case, is a manifestation of acute dystonia due to haloperidol.
   - Acute dystonia can be treated either with benztropine or diphenhydramine.

7. A 34-year-old man is brought to the emergency department due to agitation and fever. He was diagnosed with schizophreniform disorder and started on risperidone 2 weeks ago. His vital signs include a temperature of 39 F (102.2 C), a blood pressure of 175/95 mmHg, a heart rate of 130 beats/min, and a respiratory rate of 24 breaths/min. The physical examination shows diffuse muscle rigidity. Laboratory studies reveal myoglobinuria and creatine kinase 3,000 U/L (ref: 22 U/L - 198 U/L). The patient is given lorazepam. Which additional medication should be administered to this patient?

   - **Dantrolene should be administered to this patient.**
   - This young man presents with agitation and fever.
   - He was diagnosed with schizophreniform disorder and started on risperidone 2 weeks ago.
   - He has a fever of 39 C, a high blood pressure of 175/95 mmHg, tachycardia with the heart rate of 130 beats/min, and a respiratory rate of 24 breaths/min.
   - These indicate autonomic instability.
   - The physical examination shows diffuse muscle rigidity, also known as lead-pipe rigidity.
   - Laboratory studies reveal myoglobinuria and severely elevated creatine kinase at 3,000 U/L.
   - Altered mental status, autonomic instability and lead-pipe rigidity along with myoglobinuria indicates neuroleptic malignant syndrome.
   - Although neuroleptic malignant syndrome is more likely to develop with typical antipsychotics, the atypical ones, like risperidone, can also cause this condition.
   - Patients are typically given benzodiazepines to treat autonomic instability and agitation.
   - In order to treat lead-pipe rigidity, patients should also be given dantrolene to prevent exacerbation of rhabdomyolysis and subsequent acute kidney injury.
   - Now let's briefly talk about how to differentiate neuroleptic malignant syndrome from serotonin syndrome.
   - This is a high-yield distinction for both USMLE Step 1 and USMLE Step 2 CK.
   - While neuroleptic malignant syndrome is usually caused by antipsychotics, serotonin syndrome is usually caused by combination of serotonergic drugs.
   - Additionally, neuroleptic malignant syndrome is characterized by lead-pipe rigidity while serotonin syndrome presents with hyperreflexia and clonus.

REVIEW QUESTIONS

8. A 23-year-old woman is brought to the emergency department by her sister who says she has been acting "very strange." The patient is exhibiting tangential speech and says that she is talking to the "little man sitting on her shoulder." Her appearance is disheveled and she smells like she has not bathed for many days. Her sister reports that the patient has always been a little "weird," but started hearing voices and stopped taking care of herself about a year ago. She is bringing her sister to the ED because the patient quit her job, saying "the little man" told her to. What is the most likely diagnosis?

    A. Schizoaffective disorder
    B. Brief psychotic episode
    C. Schizophreniform disorder
    D. Schizophrenia
    E. Schizotypal personality disorder

- **The correct answer is D.**
- The patient exhibits multiple symptoms of a psychotic disorder including tangential speech, hallucinations, disheveled appearance, and quitting her job based.
- These symptoms could point to many different disorders, but the key here is the duration.
- The patient has been hearing voices and has not kept up her appearance for about a year.
- This length and combination of symptoms show schizophrenia.
- From the table, recall that patients must have symptoms for at least 6 months in order to make a diagnosis of schizophrenia.
- In order for it to be schizoaffective disorder the question would have had to have mentioned mood disorder symptoms such as a manic episode or depression and this was not mentioned so A is incorrect.
- Brief psychotic episode lasts for less than one month so B is incorrect.
- Schizophreniform disorder is like schizophrenia but lasts less than 6 months so C is wrong.
- Schizotypal Personality Disorder is a chronic disorder that usually presents in childhood or adulthood with less specific symptoms so E is wrong.

Psychiatry | Section 10: Dissociative Disorders

I. Dissociative Disorders
   A. Dissociation: mental impairment or disruption that results in a disconnected level of consciousness (e.g. thoughts, memories, identity, perception)
   B. Orientation to person, place, time, and reality is intact (disrupted in psychotic disorders)
   C. Associated with depression, PTSD, and childhood trauma

II. Depersonalization/Derealization Disorder
   A. Depersonalization is a persistent feeling of separation or disassociation from one's self
   B. Derealization is a persistent feeling of separation from one's environment or the outside world

III. Signs and Symptoms
   A. Flat affect
   B. Automation
   C. Feeling "in a cloud"
   D. Sense of being an outside observer of one's own mental process
   E. Intact reality testing

IV. Dissociative Amnesia
   A. Exposure to severe trauma or stress, followed by the inability to recall important personal information
   B. Associated with loss of autobiographical memory
   C. Not explained by another cause
   D. Can be reversible

V. Dissociative Amnesia vs Repression
   A. Example of dissociative amnesia:
      1. Woman is sexually assaulted in a parking garage
      2. Cannot remember the assault and CANNOT remember home address and where she works
   B. Example of repression:
      1. Woman is sexually assaulted in a parking garage
      2. Cannot remember her the assault, but CAN remember home address and where she works

VI. Dissociative Amnesia: Signs and Symptoms
   A. History of traumatic event
      1. Child abuse
      2. Sex trafficking
      3. Military combat
   B. Large groups of memories and perceptions become unavailable, not single memories, thoughts, or emotions
   C. Normal cognitive function

VII. Dissociative Fugue
   A. Characterized by unexpected wandering or travel in a dissociated state
   B. Example:
      1. A man going through a difficult divorce goes missing
      2. He is found weeks later working at a restaurant one state away
      3. He has no memory of divorce or aspects of his prior life

Disorder	Key Features	Symptoms	Comorbidities	Treatment
Depersonalization/ derealization disorder	Persistence or recurrence of depersonalization and/or derealization	Flat affect, feeling "in a cloud", automation, dreamlike experiences, intact reality testing	Depression, anxiety, OCD, avoidant personality disorder, borderline personality disorder	Psychotherapy
Dissociative amnesia	Exposure to severe trauma or stress, followed by the inability to recall important personal information	Dramatic, profound loss of memory for personal history and amnesia for personal identity	History of trauma including sexual abuse, military combat, or natural disasters; depression, substance use disorder, PTSD	Psychotherapy
Dissociative fugue	Characterized by unexpected wandering or travel in a dissociated state	Patient has unplanned traveling or wandering, inability to recall past events, loss of memory of identity	History of trauma including sexual abuse, military combat, or natural disasters; depression, substance use disorder, PTSD	Psychotherapy
Dissociative identity disorder	Involves the presence of two or more distinct personalities; formally known as multiple personality disorder	Problems with daily function, suicidal ideations, hallucinations, gaps in memories	History of trauma, PTSD, depression, substance abuse, somatoform conditions, personality disorders	Psychotherapy

TABLE 19.1.10 - Dissociative Disorders

VIII. Dissociative Identity Disorder
   A. The presence of two or more distinct identities or personality states
   B. Formerly known as multiple personality disorder
   C. More common in women

IX. Dissociative Identity Disorder: Signs and Symptoms
   A. Significant distress in the way a person functions
   B. Physical symptoms that cannot be explained by another condition
   C. Suicidal ideation
   D. Auditory hallucinations
   E. Gaps in memory

REVIEW QUESTIONS

1. A 35-year-old woman presents to the physician with her daughter reporting worsening "memory gaps." When she starts washing dishes, she commonly ends up in a car dressed like a teenager without a memory of getting into a car. She has a past medical history of transient global amnesia after a car accident. Her daughter reports she acts like six different persons in a day. The vital signs are unremarkable. The physical examination reveals a young woman alert and oriented to time, place, and person. Which of the following is the most likely diagnosis in this patient?
   A. Depersonalization-derealization disorder
   B. Dissociative amnesia
   C. Dissociative fugue
   D. Dissociative identity disorder

- **The correct answer is D.**
- This woman reports the worsening "memory gaps."
- When she starts washing dishes, she commonly ends up in a car dressed like a teenager without a memory of getting into a car.
- She was previously involved in a car accident which, presumably, was a traumatic experience for her.
- Her daughter reports she acts like six different persons in a day.
- Memory gaps, variable behavioral patterns, and multiple personalities are consistent with the diagnosis of dissociative identity disorder, previously known as multiple personality disorder.
- So correct answer is Dissociative Identity Disorder.
- Option A is incorrect because depersonalization-derealization disorder is characterized by recurrent or persistent out-of-body experiences frequently described as "being in a cloud".
- These findings are absent in this patient.
- Option B is incorrect because dissociative amnesia is characterized by forgetting the core autobiographical information.
- Although this patient has a history of transient amnesia, she is currently oriented to time, place, and person.
- Finally, option C is incorrect because dissociative fugue is characterized by wandering or travel in a dissociative state.
- Although this patient commonly ends up in a car without a memory of getting into a car, this is best explained by transition from one personality state to another.

Psychiatry | Section 11: Malingering, Factitious & Somatic Disorders

Disorder	Key Features
Malingering	- Falsification or intensification of symptoms for **external gain** (e.g. money, avoidance of work) - Aware of symptoms and why symptoms are feigned - Poor compliance with medical tests and treatment - Symptoms cease after gain is obtained
Factitious disorders	Falsification or intensification of symptoms for **internal gain** (e.g. attention, receiving affection). Aware of symptoms but lack conscious awareness of why symptoms are feigned.
Factitious disorder imposed on self (Munchausen syndrome)	- Chronic disorder characterized by physical symptoms imposed on one's self (e.g. cuts, seizures) - Willing to undergo invasive procedures and tests (multiple hospital admissions) - More common in unmarried individuals, women, and healthcare workers
Factitious disorder imposed on others (Munchausen syndrome by proxy)	- Condition is caused by caregiver who inflicts symptoms on another person - More common in caregivers of children and elderly - A form of abuse
Somatic symptom and related disorders	A group of mental disorders manifested as physical symptoms (e.g. pain, weakness, fatigue). Symptoms are not intentionally feigned or produced.
Somatic symptom disorder	- Excessive anxiety over unexplained symptoms (e.g. abdominal pain, chest pain, shortness of breath) - Must last > 6 months - Treatment includes regular visits with the same physician and psychotherapy
Conversion disorder (functional neurological symptom disorder)	- Neurological deficits (e.g. blindness, paralysis, mutism) usually following a stressor - Aware of symptoms but indifferent (La belle indifference) - More common in teens, young adults, and females
Illness anxiety disorder (hypochondriasis)	- Excessive fear of having an undiagnosed medical condition despite repeated negative evaluations - Repeated evaluations lead to high health care utilization - Few or no somatic symptoms

TABLE 19.1.11 - Malingering, Factitious Disorders, and Somatic Disorders

REVIEW QUESTIONS

1. A 30-year-old female presents as a new patient with the chief complaint of abdominal pain. She reports seeing multiple other physicians who dismissed her after negative work-ups. She has had completely normal abdominal X-rays and CTs about a year ago. She also underwent cholecystectomy and appendectomy within the last two years due to similar complaints of abdominal pain. No medications or diets have worked to fix her pain, and there are no abnormalities on imaging or labs. Based on this patient's likely diagnosis, what is the most appropriate treatment plan?

- **The most appropriate treatment plan for this patient would be to schedule regular follow-ups with the same primary care physician with the emphasis on limiting unnecessary further workups.**
- This female presents as a new patient due to abdominal pain.
- She has seen multiple other physicians and has had clear workups within the last year.
- She has had these complaints for at least two years and has undergone multiple surgeries with no relief.
- Based on this patient's presentation of vague somatic complaints with no explainable cause or treatment lasting for over 6 months, she most likely has somatic symptom disorder.
- First line treatment for this condition is regularly scheduled follow-ups with the same primary care physician with the emphasis on limiting unnecessary further workups.
- If this alone is unable to control the condition then CBT and a trial of antidepressants is warranted.

2. A 32-year-old female presents to the clinic with the chief complaint of "I have breast cancer". She offers up that none of her three gynecologists have found anything out of the ordinary on breast exam or mammogram. However, she is certain that she has breast cancer because she was told growing up that her grandmother died of breast cancer, and she believes it to run in the family. She is constantly telling friends and family that she is worried about having cancer. Physical examination is completely normal with no breast masses or tenderness appreciated. Vital signs are all within the normal range. Based on this patient's presentation, what is the most likely diagnosis?

   A. Illness anxiety disorder
   B. Somatic symptom disorder
   C. Conversion disorder
   D. Malingering

- **The correct answer is A.**
- This 32-year-old female presents with concerns of breast cancer.
- She has been to three gynecologists, all of which found normal findings on breast exam and mammograms.
- The physical exam is normal. There are no masses or tenderness present. Her vitals are normal as well.
- This patient does not have any symptoms or evidence of an actual medical condition, however she is preoccupied by the worry that she has breast cancer.
- Based on this presentation, the patient has illness anxiety disorder, thus making answer choice A correct.
- Answer choice B is incorrect because in somatic symptom disorder the patient would have a somatic related complaint. In this case the patient has no symptoms just the preoccupation with having a disease.
- Answer choice C is incorrect because in conversion disorder the patient would often have an inexplicable neurologic symptom. In this case there are no neurologic symptoms present.
- Answer choice D is incorrect because in malingering the patient would be faking an illness for secondary gain. This patient is not trying to gain anything, but is rather afraid she has a significant illness.

Psychiatry | Section 12: Personality Disorders

I. Personality Disorder
   A. A rigid pattern of behaviors that cause distress → disrupt the person's ability to function normally
   B. Usually unknown to the person → difficult to engage patient in treatment (CBT)
   C. There are three clusters:
      1. A "Weird"
      2. B "Wild"
      3. C "Worried"

Cluster	Disorder	Description
A "Weird" (genetically associated with schizophrenia)	Schizoid	- Lacks interest in relationships (romantic or platonic) → little emotional expression (may be confused with autism) and voluntary social isolation
	Schizotypal	- Superstitious with odd beliefs (apart from religious beliefs), ideas of reference (normal events carry personal significance), no hallucinations, normal cognition → often described as awkward
	Paranoid	- Deep distrust of others → suspicious, often uses projection (ego defense)
B "Wild" (genetically associated with depression, bipolar and substance abuse)	Antisocial	- Lacks empathy for others → violates other's rights through criminal behavior, must be ≥ 18 years old (< 18 indicates conduct disorder) and have evidence of conduct disorder < 15 years old
	Borderline	- Fear of abandonment and lack of identity → "black and white" thinking → described as having "mood swings", often uses splitting (ego defense), impulsive, may be self-harming (e.g. cutting), show suicidality, may threaten self-harm to manipulate others or make them feel guilty (e.g. "you don't really love me, so I'm gonna go cut myself"), treat with dialectical behavioral therapy (DBT)
	Histrionic	- Craves attention → may be sexually provocative, demonstrate dramatic dress or dramatic behavior ("drama queen"), not self-harming
	Narcissistic	- Lacks empathy others → feel they are the center of the universe → grandiose, entitled (e.g. "only the best brand of peanut butter is good enough for me"), envious (e.g. "why should they have that and not me? I'm the center of the universe"), responds angrily to criticism
C "Worried" (genetically associated with anxiety disorders)	Avoidant	- Intense feelings of inadequacy → timid, overly sensitive to criticism or rejection → involuntary (undesired) social isolation
	Obsessive-compulsive	- Believes their way is the only right way → rigid and inflexible, described as "perfectionists" (ego-syntonic, unlike the ego-dystonic OCD)
	Dependent	- Low self-confidence → clingy, extreme need for support and desire to be told what to do and frequently in abusive relationships

TABLE 19.1.12 - Personality Disorders

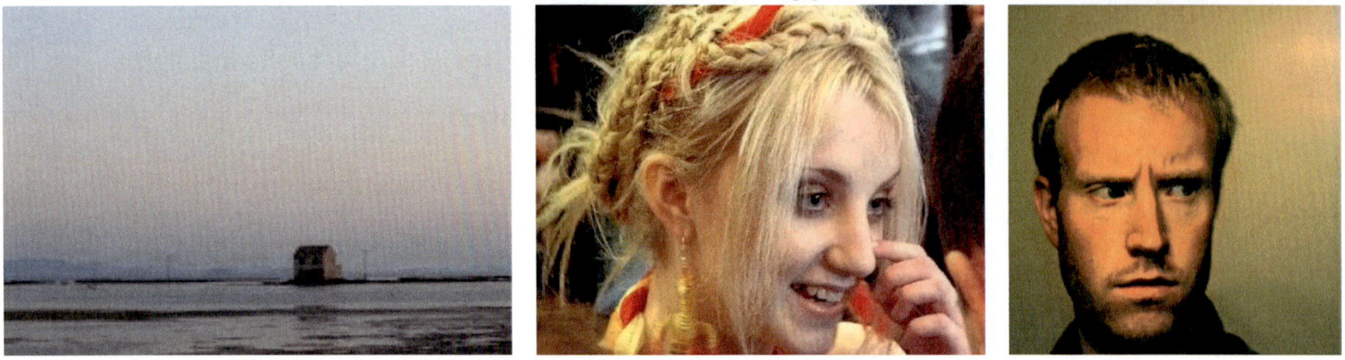

Photo Credit: Øyvind Holmstad (CC BY-SA 3.0) (left), Pat Dolan via Flickr (center), Aaron Tait via Flickr (right)

FIGURE 19.1.19 - Images Representing Schizoid, Schizotypal, and Paranoid Personality Disorders

II. Dialectical Behavioral Therapy
    A. A variation of cognitive behavioral therapy (CBT)
    B. Focused on addressing unhealthy emotions and modifying associated behaviors

III. Egosyntonic and Egodystonic
    A. Ego: balances desires (id) and rules (super-ego) → values
    B. Egosyntonic: behavior is in sync with the ego
        1. Example: obsessive-compulsive personality disorder
    C. Egodystonic: behavior conflicts with the ego
        1. Example: obsessive-compulsive disorder

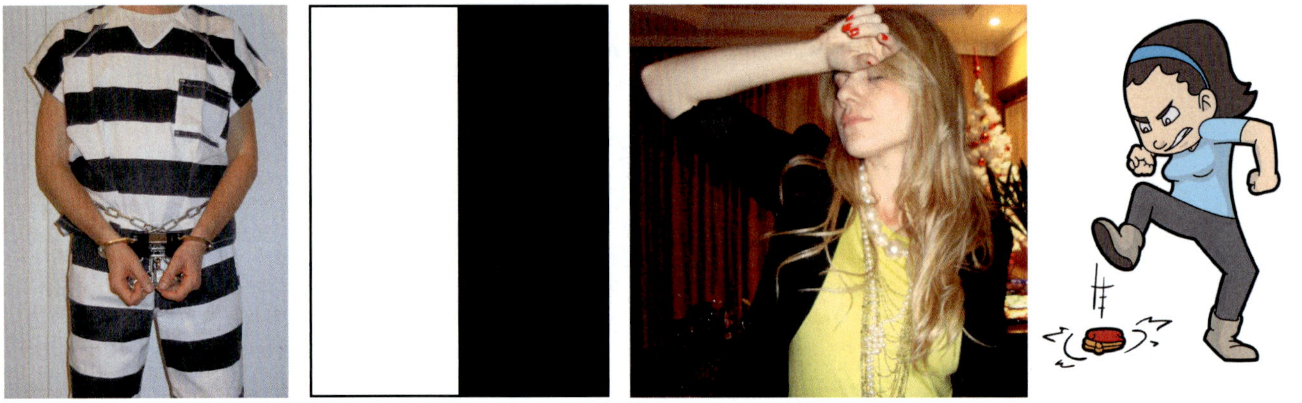

Photo Credit: Rainerzufall1234 (CC BY-SA 4.0) (left), Juliana Dacoregio (CC by 2.0) (center right), Free Clip Art [(CC BY-SA 4.0) (right)

FIGURE 19.1.20 - Images Representing Antisocial, Borderline, Histrionic and Narcissistic Personality Disorders

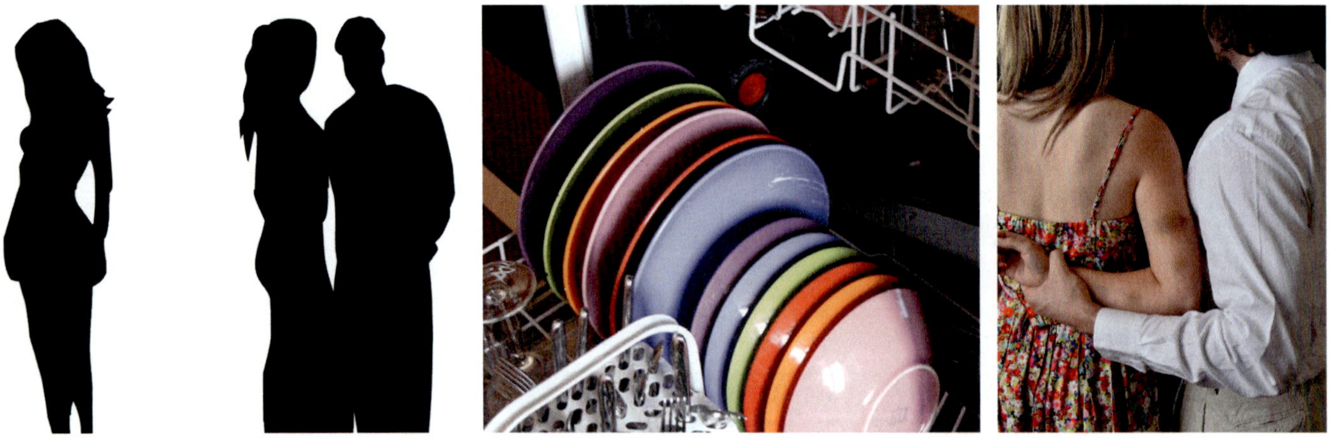

Photo Credit: ArtsyBee via Pixabay (left), andrea castelli (CC BY 2.0) (center), Zorah Olivia via Flickr (CC BY 2.0) (right)

FIGURE 19.1.21 - Images Representing Avoidant, Obsessive-Compulsive and Dependent Personality Disorders

REVIEW QUESTIONS

?

1. A 23-year-old female is presents to her family medicine doctor because she feels so depressed after her boyfriend broke up with her. She lives with roommates but reports that she doesn't have friends because everyone has "turned against" her. She has never been in trouble with the law. Her wardrobe is composed almost entirely of short skirts and fishnet tops. Assuming this patient has a personality disorder, what disorder does she most likely suffer from?

   - **This patient most likely suffers from borderline personality disorder.**
   - This patient is using very "black and white" thinking when she states that "everyone has turned against her" which is consistent with borderline personality disorder
   - Her wardrobe full of sexually provocative clothing suggests histrionic disorder, but the root of this patient's disorder is more consistent with borderline (black and white thinking), not histrionic personality disorder (craves attention)

Psychiatry | Section 13: Eating Disorders

Disorder	Definition	Diagnosis	Clinical Signs	Treatment
Anorexia nervosa	- Intense fear of weight gain - Low BMI - Two subtypes: - Restricting - Binge & purge	- Intense fear of weight gain - Low BMI (≤18.4)	- Malnutrition - Lanugo or hair loss - Amenorrhea - Osteoporosis - Hypovolemia - Hypotension - Bradycardia - Binge & purge signs possible	- Nutritional rehabilitation (watch for refeeding syndrome) - May require hospitalization - CBT - Family therapy
Bulimia nervosa	- Episodes of binge eating followed by compensatory behavior to prevent weight gain	- Binging & purging ≥ 1/ week for ≥ 3 months - Normal to high BMI (≥ 18.5)	- Binge & purge signs - Teeth erosion - Knuckle calluses - Enlarged parotids - Abdominal pain - Arrhythmia - ↓K^+, ↓Cl^-, ↑pH (serum)	- Nutritional rehabilitation - Psychotherapy - SSRIs - Avoid bupropion (seizure risk)
Binge-eating disorder	- Eating large amounts of food in a small time frame - Lack of control and distress overeating - Most common eating disorder in adults	- Binging at least 1/ week for ≥ 3 months	- Weight gain - Diabetes	- Psychotherapy with the following goals: - ↓ episodes - ↓ weight - Treat anxiety & depression
Pica	- Episodes of eating non-food substances	- Episodes for > 1 month	- Intellectual disability - Iron deficiency (sometimes zinc deficiency)	- Psychotherapy - Nutritional rehabilitation

TABLE 19.1.13 - Eating Disorders

I. Body Mass Index (BMI)
   A. BMI = Kg/m^2
      1. 18.5 - 24.9 (normal)
      2. ≤ 18.4 (low)
      3. ≥ 25 (high)

II. Restricting Subtype
   A. Disordered behavior includes:
      1. Fasting
      2. Dieting (may have strange eating rituals)
      3. Excessive exercising
   B. No binging and purging behaviors

III. Binge-Eating and Purging Subtype
   A. Binging: eating a large amount of food in a short amount of time
   B. Purging behaviors may include:
      1. Vomiting
      2. Diuretic abuse
      3. Laxative abuse
      4. Excessive exercising
   C. Different from bulimia nervosa because patient has low BMI

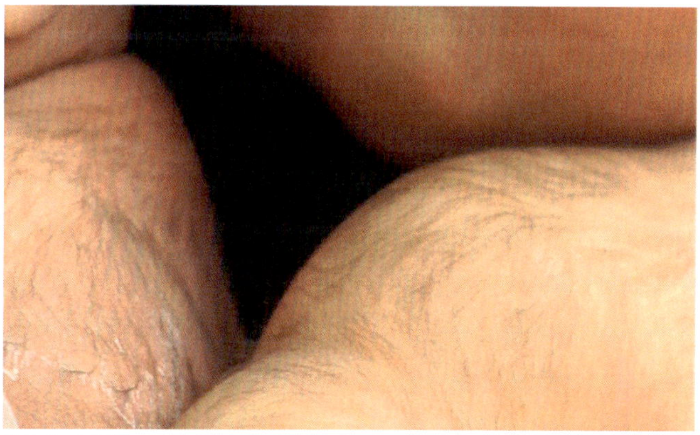

Photo Credit: Public domain via Raumka at Wikipedia

FIGURE 19.1.22 - Lanugo

IV. Refeeding Syndrome
   A. Rare, potentially fatal complication of restoring weight when refeeding patients with anorexia
   B. Starvation → ↓ glycolysis
   C. Refeeding → ↑ glycolysis → cellular uptake of K+, PO43-, Mg2+, and vitamin B1 → these substances become unavailable for other important processes → seizures, Wernicke's encephalopathy, cardiac arrest, arrhythmia, rhabdomyolysis, and respiratory failure

V. Anorexia Nervosa: Treatment
   A. Olanzapine for refractory cases
   B. Indications for hospitalization:
      1. BMI <14 Kg/m2 or <70% of ideal body weight
      2. Bradycardia; hypotension; hypothermia
      3. Cardiac dysrhythmia; moderate/severe refeeding syndrome
      4. Serious complication of malnutrition (e.g. hypoglycemia, syncope, seizures, liver or cardiac failure)

VI. Metabolic Alterations with Purging
   A. Vomiting → ↓ K^+, ↓ Cl^-, ↑ serum pH
      1. Loss of Cl^- in vomit (and H^+)
      2. Fluid loss → aldosterone (RAAS) → K^+ excretion and HCO_3^- recovery
   B. Diuretics → ↓ K^+, ↓ Cl^-, ↑ serum pH
   C. Loss of Cl^- in the urine (and K^+)
   D. Fluid loss → aldosterone (RAAS) → K^+ excretion and HCO_3^- recovery
      1. If interested, see this article for more details: Mehler PS, Walsh K. Electrolyte and acid-base abnormalities associated with purging behaviors. The International journal of eating disorders 2016; 49:311-318.
   E. Laxatives/diarrhea → ↓ K^+, ↑ Cl^-, ↓ serum pH
      1. HCO_3^- and K^+ lost in stool
      2. Water loss with little Cl^- loss → ↑ Cl concentration
   F. Laxatives (rare presentation) → ↓ K^+, ↓ Cl^-, ↑ serum pH
      1. If interested, see this article for more details: Michael Emmett, MD, Biff F Palmer, MD. Acid-base and electrolyte abnormalities with diarrhea. UpToDate inc. https://www.uptodate.com (Accessed on June 28, 2019)

VII. Binge-Eating Disorder: Treatment
   A. Cognitive behavioral therapy
   B. Pharmacotherapy:
      1. SSRIs (e.g. sertraline)
      2. Lisdexamfetamine
      3. Topiramate

REVIEW QUESTIONS ?

1. A 20-year-old girl is being treated for anorexia and she experiences 3 seizures. She has never had seizures in the past. Her seizures may be caused by low levels of what substance(s)?
   - **This patient's seizures may be caused by low levels of magnesium and phosphate.**
   - Part of this question assumes that this patient has refeeding syndrome as a result of their anexoria.
   - In refeeding syndrome, there are two substances, that if low, tend to cause seizures. These two substances are magnesium and phosphate.

REVIEW QUESTIONS

2. An 18-year-old woman is brought to the physician by her mother due to poor eating habits. She avoids eating because she thinks she is obese. Her BMI is 17 kg/m2 (18.5 kg/m2 - 24.9 kg/m2). Her vital signs include a temperature of 36 C (96.8 F), a blood pressure of 100/80 mmHg, a heart rate of 88 beats/min, and a respiratory rate of 14 breaths/min. The physical examination reveals thin hair shafts on the back. Her serum blood glucose is 50 mg/dL (70 mg/dL - 110 mg/dL). Which factor is the most likely indication for hospitalization of this patient?

- **The factor that is the most likely indication for hospitalization for this patient is hypoglycemia.**
- This young woman avoids eating because she thinks she is obese.
- Her BMI is low at 17 kg/m2.
- Distorted body image, restricted eating, and lower than normal BMI suggest the diagnosis of anorexia nervosa.
- The physical examination reveals thin hair shafts on the back.
- This sign is known as lanugo hair.
- Her serum blood glucose is low at 50 mg/dL indicating hypoglycemia.
- Hypoglycemia is one of the indications for hospitalization of anorexic patients.

3. A 32-year-old woman comes to the physician due to fatigue and trouble sleeping. She says her eating habits significantly affect her mood. She has episodes of excessive eating followed by strenuous exercise and occasional laxative use. Her BMI is 26 kg/m2 (18.5 kg/m2 - 24.9 kg/m2). She is diagnosed with bulimia nervosa and different treatment options, including medications, are discussed with her. Which class of antidepressants is indicated in this patient?

- **SSRIs is the class of antidepressants that are indicated in this patient.**
- This woman presents with fatigue and trouble sleeping.
- She says her eating habits significantly affect her mood.
- She has episodes of excessive eating followed by strenuous exercise and occasional laxative use.
- This behavioral pattern is known as binge-eating and purging.
- Her BMI is 26 kg/m2 which is slightly high.
- She is diagnosed with bulimia nervosa and different treatment options, including medications, are discussed with her.
- The antidepressants which are usually used in patients with bulimia nervosa are selective serotonin reuptake inhibitors. (10 second pause for artist: write: "SSRIs")
- However, the antidepressant that should be avoided In patients with bulimia nervosa is bupropion.
- This is because bupropion decreases seizure threshold and can induce a seizure in a bulimic patient with electrolyte disturbances.

4. A 28-year-old man comes to the physician on a follow-up visit. He has had episodes of excessive eating for the past 6 months. He feels he cannot stop eating at that time. Although he feels remorseful afterwards, he does not engage in exercise. His BMI is 42 kg/m2 (18.5 kg/m2 - 24.9 kg/m2). He was prescribed sertraline 6 weeks ago but it did not work. What are the other two drugs that can be used to treat this patient's condition?

- **Two other drugs that can be used to treat this patient are two SSRIs: lisdexamfetamine and topiramate.**
- This man has had episodes of excessive eating for the past 6 months.
- He feels he cannot stop eating at that time.
- This description is consistent with binge-eating episodes.
- Although he feels remorseful afterwards, he does not engage in exercise.
- His BMI is severely high at 42 kg/m2.
- Binge-eating episodes without purging and high BMI are consistent with binge-eating disorder.
- He was prescribed sertraline 6 weeks ago but it did not work.
- The other two drugs that can be used to treat binge-eating disorder are lisdexamfetamine and topiramate.

Psychiatry | Section 14: Sex-Related Disorders

I. Sex-Related Conditions
   A. Gender dysphoria and transgender
   B. Transvestism
   C. Sexual dysfunction
      1. Desire
      2. Arousal
      3. Orgasm
      4. Pain

II. Gender Dysphoria
   A. Significant distress or discomfort that occurs when a person experiences incongruence between their sexual identification and external sexual anatomy at birth
   B. Lasts for > 6 months
   C. Individuals may seek surgery or hormone therapy to live as another gender

III. Transgender
   A. Individual who desires to be a different gender and makes lifestyle changes to match that gender
   B. May undergo surgery or hormonal therapy to transition to desired gender

IV. Transvestism
   A. A person who derives pleasure from dressing in clothing typically associated with the opposite sex
   B. Mnemonic: "TransVESTite wears a VEST"

V. Sexual Dysfunction
   A. Sexual desire disorders: hypoactive or sexual aversion (male or female)
   B. Sexual arousal disorders: erectile dysfunction (male)
      1. Mnemonic for causes of erectile dysfunction: "PENIS"
   C. Orgasmic disorders: anorgasmia (male or female), premature ejaculation (male)
   D. Sexual pain disorders: vaginismus or dyspareunia (female)

VI. Differential Diagnosis for Erectile Dysfunction
   A. "PENIS"
      1. Psychological (if nighttime erections still occur)
      2. Endocrine (diabetes, low testosterone)
      3. Neurogenic (spinal cord injury)
      4. Insufficient blood flow (atherosclerosis)
      5. Substances (ethanol)

VII. Management of Erectile Dysfunction
   A. Detailed history, physical examination, and laboratory tests
   B. Phallography: helps differentiate between organic and psychological causes
   C. First line therapy: phosphodiesterase-5 inhibitors

VIII. Sexual Dysfunction
   A. Orgasmic disorders: anorgasmia (male or female), premature ejaculation (male)
      1. Premature ejaculation are treated with SSRIs and psychotherapy
   B. Sexual pain disorders: vaginismus or dyspareunia (female)

REVIEW QUESTIONS

1. A 37-year-old male presents to the office due to recent problems with erections. He states he has issues with both achieving and maintaining an erection in the bedroom with his wife. He has no past medical history and is in good health. He states he and his wife have a good marriage with 3 children, but he has been stressed within the last month at work due to his boss treating him poorly. What could the patient be asked to best confirm the reason for his recent erectile dysfunction?
   - **The best question to help confirm this diagnosis is to ask if he still has night time or early morning erections.**
   - This patient presents with erectile dysfunction and has issues both achieving and maintaining erections.
   - He is in good health and he and his wife have a good marriage.
   - However, he has been stressed within the last month at work due to poor treatment from his boss.
   - Based on the symptoms and recent increase in stress, this patient likely has psychogenic erectile dysfunction.
   - The best question to help confirm this diagnosis is to ask if he still has night time or early morning erections.
   - If a patient still has morning or night erections, then they are capable of achieving erection, but cannot do it during sexual interactions due to a pschogenic cause.

REVIEW QUESTIONS

2. A 29-year-old heterosexual female presents with concerns for sexual dysfunction. She has a normal sex drive and a healthy relationship with her husband. Currently, she can be aroused and has been able to orgasm in the past. However, since the natural birth of her third child 5 months ago, she and her husband have only had sexual intercourse once. Since that one experience, she has avoided sex. What is most likely contributing to her aversion to sexual intercourse?

- **The most likely contribution to her aversion to sexual intercourse is pain.**
- The categories of sexual dysfunction problems with desire are problems with arousal, orgasm, or pain.
- The most likely issue here is pain.
- Since her sex drive is normal, there is not any apparent problem with desire.
- The patient can also still be aroused and has orgasms in the past.
- The only thing that's changed recently is that she had a baby and had a bad experience with sex afterwards.
- Since she has a good relationship with her husband and its unlikely that she just decided she's not going to have sex with her husband just because she didn't orgasm the last time she engaged in sex, this leads to the conclusion that the most logical reason as to why the patient is adverse to sexual intercourse is pain.

3. A 27-year old male presents to the clinic with a two-month history of premature ejaculation. He states that he only recently decided to begin having sex after breaking up with a longterm girlfriend with whom he had planned on waiting until marriage. However, it has been difficult because everytime he begins having vaginal intercourse, he ejaculates within a minute. This causing tension between him and the women he is having intercourse with, and it makes him feel upset and judged. What is the best treatment option for this patient?

   A. Sildenafil
   B. Hormone Therapy
   C. Selegiline
   D. Sertraline

- **The correct answer is D.**
- This patient presents due to a two-month history of premature ejactulation.
- He only recently decided to begin having sex and everytime he begins vaginal intercourse, he ejaculates within a minute.
- This issue has been causing tension between him and his sexual partner as well as making him feel upset and judged.
- This patient meets the diagnostic criteria for premature ejaculation since it occurs within an minute and is causing some psychological distress in his life.
- The treatment for premature ejactulation is SSRIs thus making answer choice D correct.
- Let's discuss other answer choices.
- Answer choice A is incorrect because sildenafil is a phosphodiesterase-5 inhibitor used to treat erectile dysfunction.
- Answer choice B is incorrect because hormone therapy may be used in a patient with gender dysphoria not premature ejaculation.
- Answer choice C is incorrect because selegiline is an MAO inhibitor not an SSRI.

Psychiatry | Section 15: Sleep Disorders

I. Sleep Stages
   A. Awake (eyes open)
   B. Awake (eyes closed)
   C. Non-REM sleep
      1. Stage N1
      2. Stage N2
      3. Stage N3
   D. REM sleep (increases during the night)

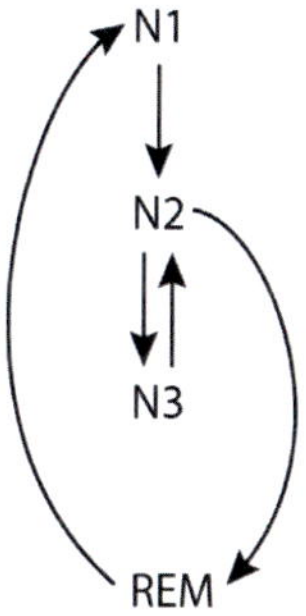

FIGURE 19.1.23 - Sequence of Sleep Stages

II. Awake
   A. Eyes open - most alert or concentrating
      1. Beta waves
   B. Eyes closed
      1. Alpha waves

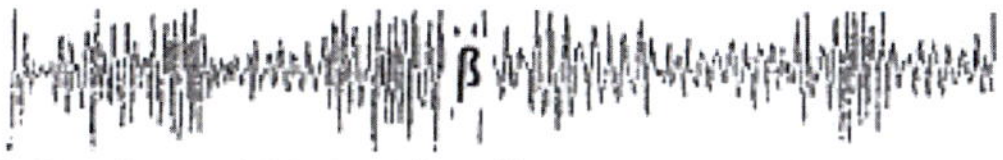

FIGURE 19.1.24 - Beta Waves

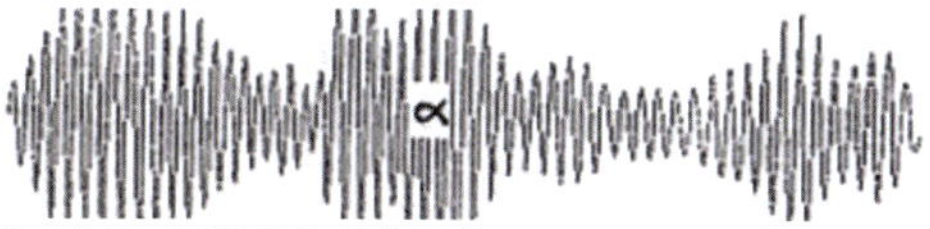

FIGURE 19.1.25 - Alpha Waves

III. Non-REM Sleep
   A. Stage N1
      1. Transition from awake to sleep - easily awakened
      2. Least amount of sleep time spent in N1
      3. Hypnagogic hallucinations
      4. Theta waves

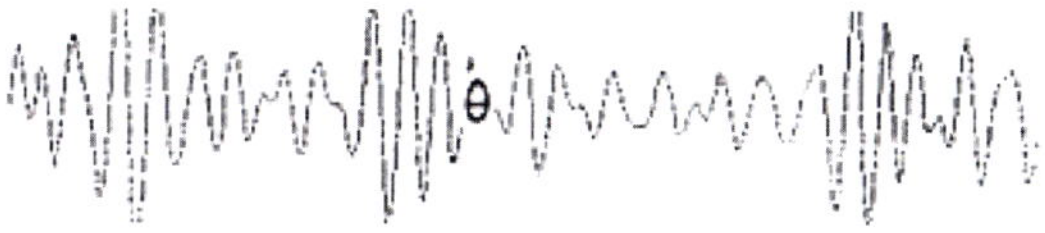

FIGURE 19.1.26 - Theta Waves

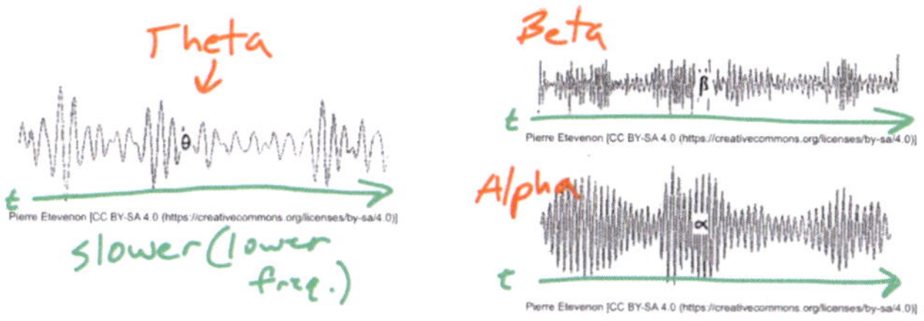

IV. Non-REM Sleep
   A. Stage N2
      1. Largest amount of sleep time spent in this stage - deeper sleep
      2. Bruxism - tooth grinding ("2 for tooth")
      3. Theta waves with sleep spindles and K complexes

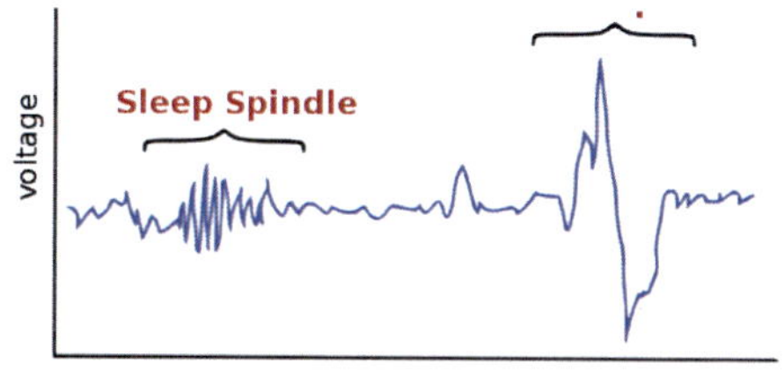

FIGURE 19.1.27 - Sleep Spindles and K Complexes

V. Non-REM Sleep
   A. Stage N3
      1. Slow wave sleep
      2. Sleepwalking, night terrors, bedwetting
      3. Delta waves
      4. Memory hook: Pee and flee in N3

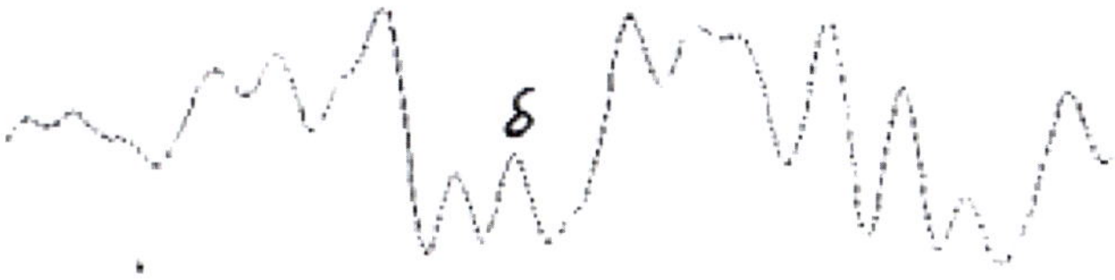

FIGURE 19.1.28 - Delta Waves

VI. REM Sleep
   A. Increases in frequency and duration throughout the night
   B. Paradoxical sleep with EEG beta waves - same as awake (eyes open)
   C. Dreaming and nightmares that can be REMembered
   D. May be involved in memory processing
   E. Paramedian pontine reticular formation causes eye movements
   F. Bodily changes:
      1. Increased oxygen use by the brain
      2. Increased acetylcholine
      3. Penile/clitoral swelling
      4. Loss of muscle tone
      5. Variable blood pressure/pulse
   G. Drugs that decrease REM sleep and N3 Sleep
      1. Alcohol
      2. Benzodiazepines
      3. Barbiturates
   H. NE decreases only REM

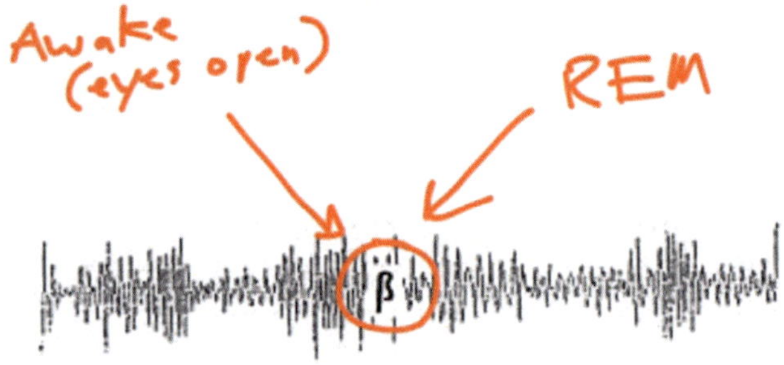

FIGURE 19.1.29 - Memory Hooks for EEG Findings

VII. Memory Hook for EEG Findings
  A. BATS Drink Blood
  B. Beta - Eyes Open
  C. Alpha - Eyes Closed
  D. Theta - N1
  E. Sleep Spindle - N2
  F. Delta - N3
  G. Beta - REM

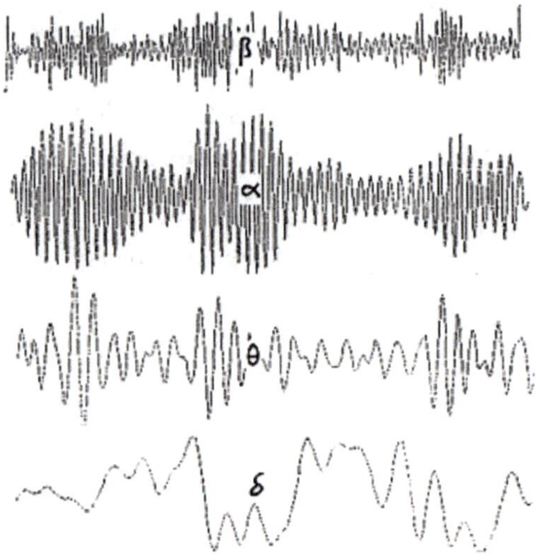

FIGURE 19.1.30 - Sleep Spindles and K Complexes

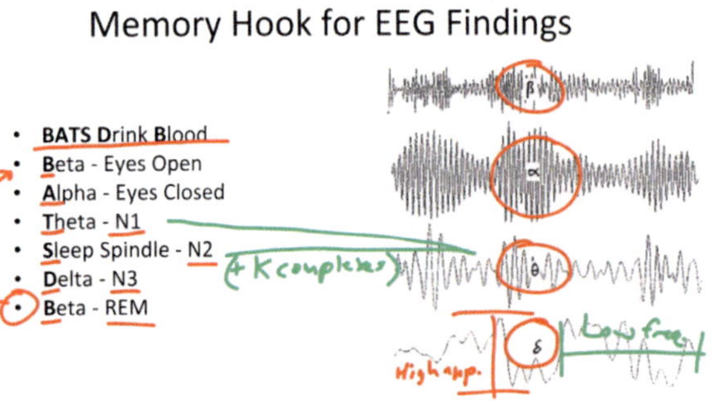

FIGURE 19.1.31 - Memory Hooks for EEG Findings

VIII. Sleep Changes
  A. Elderly
    1. Decreased N3 and REM, as well as total sleep time
    2. Increased time to REM (↑ REM latency)
    3. Wake up more often during the night → daytime napping
  B. Depression
    1. Decreased N3 and increased REM
    2. Decreased time to REM (↓ REM latency)
    3. Nighttime and early morning awakening

IX. Sleep Terror Disorder
  A. Periods of partial awakening from sleep caused by feelings of terror accompanied with screaming
  B. Occurs in N3 (not remembered)
    1. Contrast to nightmares (REM sleep; remembered)
  C. Children
  D. Emotional stress, fever, lack of sleep
  E. Self-limiting (benzodiazepines)

X. Enuresis
  A. Bedwetting - greater than 2 times per week for 3 months in a person older than 5 years old
  B. Primary and secondary enuresis
  C. Treatment:
    1. Behavioral modification (e.g. scheduled voids, nighttime fluid restriction)
    2. Alarm
    3. Oral desmopressin (better than imipramine which has more side effects)

XI. Narcolepsy
  A. Excessive daytime sleepiness more than 3 times per week for 3 months
    1. Not tired upon awakening, yet experience daytime sleepiness
    2. Caused by decreased hypocretin (orexin) 1 and 2 production; leads to circadian rhythm disruptions
  B. Associated with:
    1. Sleep episodes with rapid fall into REM
    2. Cataplexy (strong stimulation → loss of muscle tone)
    3. Hypnagogic and hypnopompic hallucinations
  C. Treatment:
    1. Daytime stimulants (modafinil) and or nighttime sodium oxybate

XII. Nightmare Disorder
  A. Nightmares are disturbing dreams that awakens from sleep
  B. Nightmare disorder: repetitive nightmares with disruption of sleep and impairment of day-to-day activities
    1. Considered as REM-related sleep disorder
  C. Most common risk factor is post traumatic stress disorder
  D. Clinical features:
    1. Repetitive episodes of nightmares, typically during the second half of night
    2. Patient is alert when awakening
    3. Full memory of nightmare content
    4. Patient is consolable

E. Diagnosis:
   1. Clinical diagnosis
   2. Polysomnography to rule out other sleep disorders (e.g. OSA)
F. Treatment:
   1. Mild cases: reassurance
   2. Psychotherapy: imagery rehearsal therapy
   3. Associated PTSD: antidepressants or prazosin

XIII. REM Sleep Behavior Disorder
A. Mostly a disorder of elderly men
B. Characteristic feature: no loss of muscle tone
C. Patient physically act out violent dreams and fall off or cause harm to self or others
D. Patient clearly remembers the dream after awakening (vs. sleepwalking disorder)
E. Risk factors:
   1. Neurodegenerative disorders (e.g. Parkinson's disease, Lewy body dementia)
   2. Psychiatric drugs, narcolepsy
F. Treatment:
   1. Melatonin receptor agonist, benzodiazepines
   2. Remove offending agent and secure patient safety

REVIEW QUESTIONS

1. An 8-year-old boy is brought to the clinic because his mother says he is always sleeping. She states that he sleeps through the night, but then can seemingly fall asleep anywhere throughout the day. She is worried he is not getting restful sleep at night since he is taking so many naps during the day. When talking to the patient, he says he has weird dreams when he starts to sleep and sometimes does not know if he is dreaming or awake. What is most likely deficient in this patient?
   - **The most likely deficient in this patient is hypocretin, or orexin 1 & 2.**
   - This patient presents due to always sleeping and being able to fall asleep anywhere throughout the day.
   - The patient also notes that he sometimes has weird dreamlike hallucinations as he is going to sleep.
   - These dreamlike hallucinations are hypnagogic hallucinations which occur when going to sleep; they are also a feature of narcolepsy which this child most likely has.
   - In narcolepsy there is decreased hypocretin, or orexin 1 & 2.
   - Also note that orexin antagonists are some of the newer medications currently in use for insomnia in patients who have trouble going to sleep.

2. A 79-year-old man comes into the clinic due to restless sleeping. His wife constantly tells him that he moves around too much during the night and occasionally hits or kicks her accidentally. Usually when his wife awakens him, he is able to recall violent dreams. He says the dreams are not nightmares and he does not awake scared; the dreams just usually involve a lot of moving around. He states he does not remember doing this as a younger man. He also claims to get enough sleep to where he is not tired throughout the day. What is the most common risk factor for this patient's likely diagnosis?
   A. PTSD diagnosis
   B. Hypocretin deficiency
   C. Parkinson's disease
   D. Benzodiazepine use

- **The correct answer is C.**
- This elderly man presents with restless sleeping and accidental injury to his bed partner.
- On awakening he is able to recall the dreams which are not nightmares.
- He is also not tired throughout the day and did not have this issue all of his life.
- This patient most likely has a diagnosis of REM sleep behavior disorder which is associated with neurodegenerative disorders like Parkinson's disease or the dementias.
- Answer choice A is incorrect because PTSD is associated with nightmare disorder that presents with repetitive nightmares impairing sleep and daily function which this patient does not have.
- Additionally in nightmare disorder the patient would have loss of muscle tone and not act out any dreams.
- Answer choice B is incorrect because Hypocretin deficiency is associated with narcolepsy which presents as rapidly entering REM sleep during the day & night. Also this would present at a much younger age than this patient's.
- Answer choice D is incorrect because benzodiazepine use actually decreases REM sleep and would be a treatment option for this patient's condition not a risk factor.

Psychiatry | Section 16: Substance Use Disorder & Stages of Change

I. Substance Use Disorder
   A. Maladaptive pattern of substance use for ≥1 year with ≥2 of the following:
      1. Withdrawal
      2. Excessive use
      3. Inability to cut down
      4. Continued use despite awareness of harm
      5. Tolerance
      6. Hazardous (≥1 episode)
      7. Activities give up for substance use
      8. Time consuming
      9. Cravings
      10. Obligations
      11. Personal problems

II. Substance Use Disorder: Mnemonic
   A. "WE couldn't stop harming THAT COP for over a year"

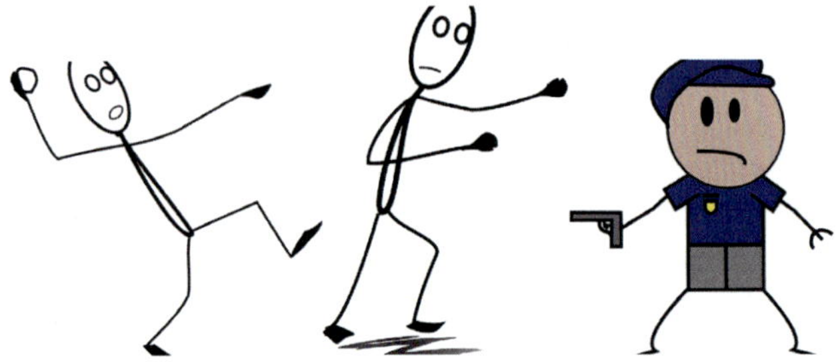

FIGURE 19.1.32 - Substance Use Disorder Mnemonic

   B. Withdrawal symptoms
   C. Excessive use; longer amount of time/higher dose than intended
   D. "Couldn't stop": inability to cut down despite a persistent desire
   E. "Harming": continued use despite awareness of harm
   F. Tolerance
   G. Hazardous: dangerous actions (≥ 1; eg, needle sharing/drunk driving)
   H. Activities: social, recreational, and occupational activities given up
   I. Time consuming - acquiring, using, recovering
   J. Cravings
   K. Obligations: failure to fulfill duties at home, school, and work
   L. Personal problems: recurrent interpersonal or social problems

III. Substance-Induced Disorders
   A. Intoxication: transient condition altering patient's consciousness, perception, behaviour, and/or affect with recent ingestion of substance
   B. Withdrawal: physiological, cognitive and behavioural changes after the sudden cessation of substance use
   C. Substance induced psychiatric disorder: occurs within 1 month of substance use and doesn't qualify for independent mental disorder

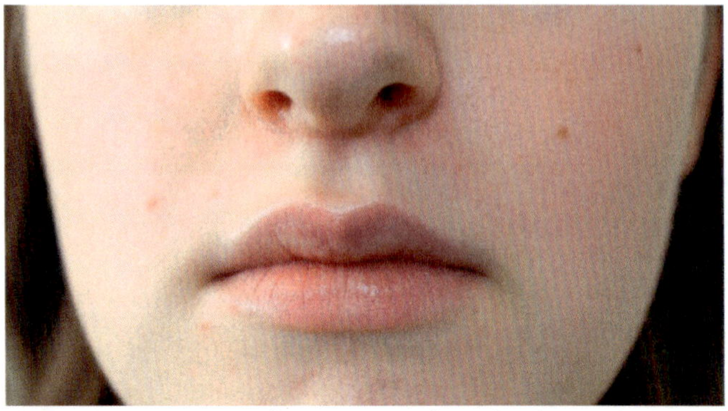

FIGURE 19.1.33 - Perioral Dermatitis

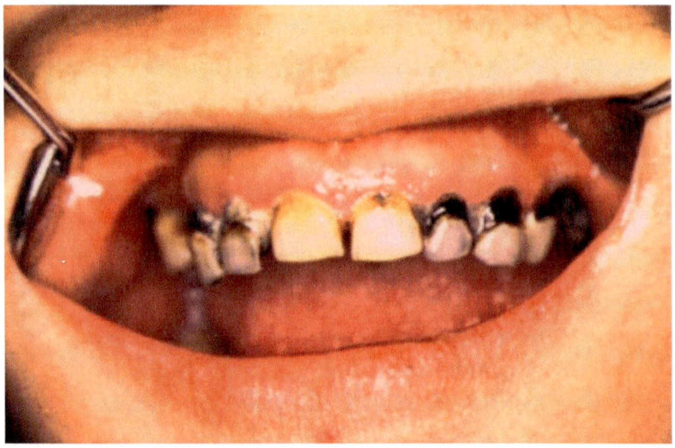

FIGURE 19.1.34 - Meth Mouth

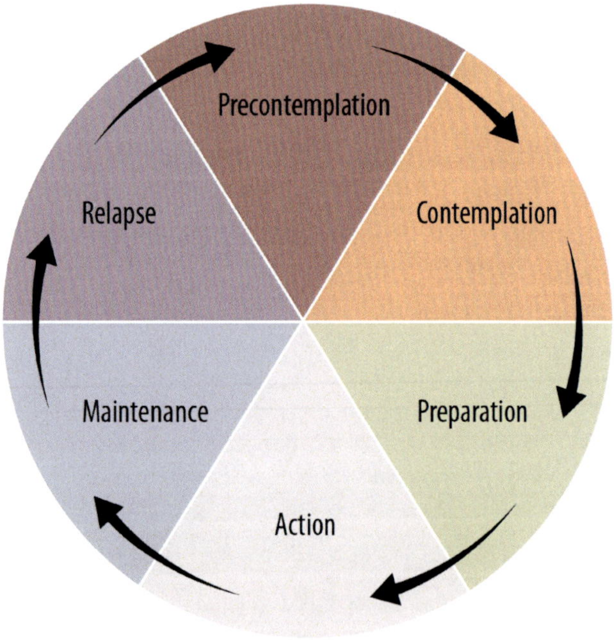

FIGURE 19.1.35 - Stages of Change

Substance	Intoxication Symptoms	Treatment
Alcohol	Euphoria, impaired judgment, inattention, slurred speech, ataxia	Supportive (e.g. fluids), thiamine
Benzodiazepines	Somnolence, lethargy, ataxia, slurred speech, respiratory depressions	Supportive treatment
Opioids	Altered mental status, miosis, constipation, hypothermia, bradycardia, seizures, respiratory depression	Supportive treatment, naloxone, naltrexone
Inhalants	Headache, slurred speech, disorientation, tremors, altered gait, stomach cramps, coughing, arrhythmia, glue sniffer's rash, anorexia and neurocognitive dysfunction in chronic use	Supportive treatment, intubation
Cocaine	Euphoria, tachycardia, angina, mydriasis, hallucinations, perforated nasal septum, weight loss	Supportive treatment, benzodiazepines
Methamphetamine	Hypertension, tachycardia, diaphoresis, hyperthermia, teeth grinding, agitation, psychosis, "meth mouth" in chronic use	Supportive treatment, benzodiazepines
PCP	Aggressive behaviours, nystagmus, ataxia, dissociation, tachycardia, hypertension, hyperthermia	Supportive treatment, benzodiazepines, anti-psychotics
MDMA	Tachycardia, hypertension, bruxism, hyponatremia, serotonin syndrome	Supportive treatment, fluid restriction, benzodiazepines, anti-psychotics
LSD	Psychosis, depersonalization, flashbacks, visual hallucinations	Supportive treatment, benzodiazepines, anti-psychotics
Cannabis	Euphoria, impaired reaction time and concentration, conjunctival injection, dry mouth, increased appetite	Symptomatic treatment

TABLE 19.1.14 - Substances, Intoxication Symptoms and Treatment

IV. Stages of Change

A. Stage1: Precontemplation. The patient hasn't even thought about the problem. They don't recognize that there is a problem.

B. Stage 2: Contemplation and this is when the patient notices the problem but is still unwilling to change.

C. Stage 3: Preparation and this is when the patient is actually beginning to make changes. In this stage the patient may make a plan to quit, obtain resources necessary to facilitate change, or inform friends and family about the change so that support is in place as needed.

D. Stage 4: Action. In this stage the patient actually attempts to stops using. An example of this is includes a patient who may go to a detox center or just stop using.

E. Stage 5: Maintenance. This is when the patient has achieved some success with abstinence and is now upholding a standard of behavior.

1. If the patient is unable to stay in this maintenance stage then they relapse and the cycle starts over again.

REVIEW QUESTIONS

1. A 23-year-old female began drinking alcohol 2 years ago. She is concerned about this behavior and asks her physician if she should stop. Upon further inquiry she states that she drinks at bars about once a month with her friends. One time she drank too much and vandalized a property but felt guilty the next day. Should she be diagnosed with substance use disorder?

- **This patient should not be diagnosed with substance use disorder.**
- This patient began drinking 2 years ago which fits part of the diagnosis for substance use disorder (the individual must be using the substance for at least 1 year). However, we can't really identify 2 of the 11 possible criteria (she only drinks about once a month which is not excessive use).
- She did end up drinking too much one time and participated in vandalism but this was an isolated event.
- Therefore, we can conclude that she does NOT have substance use disorder and this is most likely normal behavior

2. A 16-year-old boy is brought to the emergency department from school due to acute confusion, staggering gait, and stomach cramps. The teacher said he seemed normal before lunch break. The physical examination shows slurred speech, tremor, and mild perioral rash. Blood alcohol level is 0 mg/dL. What is the most likely cause of this patient's presentation?

- **The most likely cause of this patient's presentation is inhalant abuse.**
- This young boy presents with acute confusion, staggering gait, and stomach cramps.
- The physical examination shows slurred speech, tremor, and mild perioral rash.
- His blood alcohol level is 0 mg/dL, making alcohol intoxication unlikely.
- These findings are consistent with inhalant abuse.
- Chronic inhalant abuse may also lead to anorexia and neurocognitive dysfunction.

3. A 32-year-old man is brought to the emergency department due to retrosternal chest pain for the past 30 minutes. His vital signs include a blood pressure of 180/120 mmHg, a heart rate of 135 beats/min, and a respiratory rate of 22 breaths/min. The physical examination reveals mydriasis and a perforated nasal septum. His BMI is 18 kg/m2 (19 kg/m2 - 25 kg/m2). What is the most likely cause of this patient's presentation?

- **The most likely cause of this patient's presentation is cocaine intoxication.**
- This young man presents with retrosternal chest pain for the past 30 minutes.
- His vital signs show severe hypertension and tachycardia.
- The physical examination reveals mydriasis and perforated nasal septum.
- His BMI is low at 18 kg/m2 suggesting possible anorexia.
- All these signs and symptoms are consistent with the acute cocaine intoxication in the context of chronic cocaine abuse.
- While acute intoxication presents with sympathetic symptoms such as hypertension, tachycardia, and mydriasis, chronic abuse is characterized by perforated septum and anorexia.
- Cocaine intoxication may mimic amphetamine intoxication.
- However, chronic amphetamine use usually results in obsessive skin picking and poor dentition that are not seen in this patient.

REVIEW QUESTIONS

4. A 41-year-old man is brought to the emergency department due to right arm pain after he physically assaulted his neighbour. It took 4 police officers to put him in the car. He is physically restrained in the emergency department due to his violent behavior. His vital signs include a blood pressure of 150/100 mmHg, and a heart rate of 125 beats/min. The physical examination shows vertical nystagmus. X-ray of his right arm reveals a humeral midshaft fracture. What is the most likely cause of this patient's presentation?

   - **The most likely cause of this patient's presentation is PCP intoxication.**
   - This man presents with right arm pain after he physically assaulted his neighbour.
   - It took 4 police officers to put him in the car.
   - He is physically restrained in the emergency department due to his violent behavior.
   - His vital signs show hypertension and tachycardia.
   - The physical examination shows vertical nystagmus.
   - All these findings suggest the use of phencyclidine, also known as PCP.
   - PCP is a hallucinogenic substance that makes abuser particularly aggressive and violent.

5. A 57-year-old man is evaluated due to fever and confusion 4 days after undergoing laparoscopic cholecystectomy due to acute cholecystitis. He feels spiders crawling under his skin. His vital signs include a temperature of 40 C (104 F), a blood pressure of 155/100 mmHg, a heart rate of 132 beats/min, and a respiratory rate of 23 breaths/min. The physical examination reveals a tremor and perspiration. CBC is normal. Blood and urine cultures are negative. What is the most likely cause of this patient's presentation?

   - **The most likely cause of this patient's presentation is delirium tremens.**
   - This middle-aged man is evaluated due to fever and confusion 4 days after undergoing laparoscopic cholecystectomy.
   - He feels spiders crawling under his skin. This phenomenon is known as a tactile hallucination.
   - His vital signs show hyperthermia, hypertension, and tachycardia.
   - The physical examination reveals tremor and perspiration.
   - All these signs indicate autonomic instability.
   - If this patient had hypotension, abnormal CBC, and positive cultures, sepsis would be the most reasonable diagnosis.
   - In contrast, he has hypertension, normal CBC, and negative cultures.
   - Therefore, the most likely cause of his presentation is delirium tremens.
   - Delirium tremens is the most severe form of alcohol intoxication that occurs 48 to 96 hours after last drink.

REVIEW QUESTIONS

6. A 43-year-old homeless man is brought to the emergency department due to diffuse body aches for the past 2 days. He also complains of frequent bowel movements and difficulty sleeping. His vital signs are significant for a heart rate of 120 beats/min. The physical examination reveals excessive tearing, runny nose, and piloerection. The patient is frequently yawning during examination. What is the most likely cause of this patient's presentation?

- **The most likely cause of this patient's presentation is opioid withdrawal.**
- This homeless man presents with diffuse body aches for the past 2 days.
- He also complains of frequent bowel movements and difficulty sleeping.
- The physical examination reveals excessive tearing and runny nose as well as piloerection.
- The patient is frequently yawning during examination.
- Diffuse body pain, diarrhea, lacrimation, rhinorrhea, piloerection and yawning are all signs and symptoms of the opioid withdrawal.

7. A 45-year-old female presents to the clinic with a 2-month history of insomnia and anxiety. During the patient interview she states that she has been using methamphetamine for the past 7 months. She is worried that the drugs are becoming a problem and wants to make goals to get help. She expresses concern about her ability to quit, but is willing to follow the physician's direction and see a psychiatrist who specializes in substance use recovery. The patient is most likely at what stage of change in overcoming addiction?

   A. Action
   B. Contemplation
   C. Precontemplation
   D. Preparation
   E. Maintenance

- **The correct answer is D.**
- This woman is in the preparation stage of change to overcome her addiction.
- She is seeing a doctor, making goals, and is willing to see a psychiatrist.
- In other words, she has made a plan to change her behavior and is willing to make steps to change.
- A is wrong because she hasn't actually stopped using and isn't a treatment center yet.
- B is wrong because the contemplative stage is more indicative of a person who knows they have a problem but doesn't want to change their behavior.
- C is wrong because this is when a patient hasn't even recognized the problem.
- This patient clearly recognizes the problem and is making plans to change.
- Finally, E is wrong because maintenance is continuing those changes for an extended period of time and this patient hasn't made changes yet.

Psychiatry | Section 17: Trauma & Stress-Related Disorders

Disorder	Description	Time	Treatment
Post-traumatic stress disorder (PTSD)	Intrusive thoughts (e.g. flashbacks, avoidance of reminders, sleep disturbances, nightmares), feelings (e.g. fear, horror, distress, dissociative symptoms) and/or behaviors (eg, avoidance of reminders, hypervigilance) following a traumatic event (e.g. abuse, military service, witnessing death)	- Symptoms must last > 1 month	- CBT - SSRIs - Venlafaxine - Prazosin to reduce nightmares
Acute stress disorder	Similar to PTSD	- Symptoms last 3 days to 1 month	- CBT
Adjustment disorder	Emotional distress (e.g. depression, anxiety) following a psychosocial stressor (e.g. loss of employment, divorce) Symptoms do not meet criteria for another psychiatric disorder	- Symptoms must occur within 3 months of the stressor - Lasts < 6 months - If > 6 months then it is GAD	- CBT - Adjunctive pharmacotherapy (e.g. zolpidem, SSRIs)

TABLE 19.1.15 - Trauma and Stress-Related Disorders

REVIEW QUESTIONS

1. A 25-year-old male presents to the physician due to difficulty sleeping from nightmares. He was physically and sexually assaulted by strangers three months ago. He moved out of the neighborhood where he was attacked. His girlfriend reports he has recently become distant and irritable. The physical examination reveals a man with poor eye contact. Cognitive behavioral therapy as well as sertraline are initiated. Which medication will most likely alleviate his night-time complaint?

   - **Prazosin, an alpha-1 agonist, will most likely alleviate this patient's night-time complaint.**
   - This young man was physically and sexually assaulted by strangers 3 months ago.
   - He complains of difficulty sleeping from nightmares. This means he is re-experiencing his traumatic event through dreams.
   - He moved out of the neighborhood where he was attacked. In other words, he avoids the stimuli associated with the event.
   - Finally, his girlfriend reports he has recently become distant and irritable.
   - Re-experience of traumatic event, avoidance of associated stimuli, and mood changes for more than 1 month suggest the diagnosis of post-traumatic stress disorder.
   - Cognitive behavioral therapy as well as sertraline is initiated.
   - Apart from these interventions, prazosin, an alpha-1 antagonist, has been specifically shown to decrease nightmares in patients with PTSD.

2. A 31-year-old police officer comes to the physician due to recent mood changes. She often finds herself shouting at her children for no reason. She also reports nightmares and disrupted sleep. Two weeks ago, she saw her colleague's car explode in the street. She quit her job after the accident. What is the best treatment option for this patient?

   - **The best treatment option for this patient is cognitive behavioral therapy.**
   - This patient presents with recent mood changes.
   - She often finds herself shouting at her children for no reason.
   - She also reports nightmares and disrupted sleep.
   - 2 weeks ago, she saw her colleague's car explode in the street. She quit her job after the accident which means she avoids the stimuli associated with the traumatic event.
   - Mood changes, disrupted sleep, and avoidance of associated stimuli for less than a month after traumatic event suggest the diagnosis of acute stress disorder.
   - The best treatment option for acute stress disorder is cognitive behavioral therapy.
   - If patient continues to have symptoms after 1 month, then she will be diagnosed with PTSD and likely need pharmacological therapy as well.

REVIEW QUESTIONS

3. A 41-year-old woman presents to the physician with low mood for the past month after getting divorced. She no longer enjoys going out for shopping with her friends. She has never had similar complaints before. Her past medical history includes sexual abuse from her childhood. She occasionally has nightmares about her traumatic childhood experience. She constantly worries about her children's education, her job, and upcoming bills. Her vital signs are unremarkable. The physical examination reveals an irritable restless woman who fidgets in her chair. Which of the following is the most likely diagnosis in this patient?

    A. PTSD
    B. Acute stress disorder
    C. Adjustment disorder
    D. Generalized anxiety disorder

- **The correct answer is C.**
- This woman presents with low mood for the past month after getting divorced.
- She no longer enjoys going out for shopping with her friends.
- This latter sign is known as anhedonia.
- She has never had similar complaints before.
- In other words, this is an acute change in her mood and functioning.
- She constantly worries about her children's education, her job, and upcoming bills.
- The physical examination reveals an irritable restless woman who fidgets in her chair.
- This patient has symptoms of both depression and anxiety.
- However, she does not fully meet criteria for major depressive disorder or generalized anxiety disorder.
- Additionally, her mood change was preceded by significant stressor, that is divorce.
- All these clues suggest the diagnosis of adjustment disorder.
- Acute mood change within 3 months of significant stressor that does not last for more than 6 months is known as adjustment disorder.
- Option A is incorrect because post-traumatic stress disorder, that is PTSD, is associated with hypervigilance, avoidance of associated stimuli, nightmares, and flashbacks.
- Although this patient was sexually abused in childhoood and has nightmares about her traumatic experience, her mood change is acute so PTSD cannot explain the other findings.
- Option B is incorrect because acute stress disorder lasts less than 1 month.
- This patient has already been having symptoms for a month.
- Finally, option D is incorrect because generalized anxiety disorder lasts more than 6 months.
- Additionally, generalized anxiety disorder is not characterized by depressive symptoms seen in this patient.

TABLES & FIGURES

Made in United States
Orlando, FL
04 November 2026

90207061R00036